CHILDHOOD
SYMPTOMS

CHILDHOOD SYMPTOMS

Every Parent's Guide to Childhood Illnesses

Edward R. Brace
John P. Pacanowski, M.D., F.A.A.P.C

Revised by Ed Weiner

A Stonesong Press Book

HarperPerennial
A Division of HarperCollins*Publishers*

HarperCollins books may be purchased for educational, business, or sales
promotional use. For information, please call or write: Special Markets
Department, HarperCollins Publishers, Inc., 10 East 53rd Street, New
York, NY 10022. Telephone: (212) 207-7528; Fax: (212) 207-7222.

Library of Congress Catalog Card Number 91-55391

ISBN 0–06–271532–1 (hc)
ISBN 0–06–273078–9 (pbk)
92 93 94 95 96 PS/RRD 10 9 8 7 6 5 4 3 2 1

Contents

Important Telephone Numbers

Poison Control Center _____
   (See page 305 for Directory of Poison-Control Centers)

Emergency Room _____

Mobile Emergency Treatment Facility _____

Police _____

Fire Department _____

Doctor _____

Druggist _____

Taxi _____

Before You Call the Doctor/Health-Care Professional:
SYMPTOM CHART/CHECKLIST

The following checklist will help you provide information to your child's doctor/health-care professional as well as afford you personal health records for your files. Keep these points in mind when you call so that the information you give the doctor/health-care professional is as thorough as possible. Feel free to photocopy this page and bring it with you to the doctor's/health-care professional's office.

● What are the symptoms? _____

_____

_____

● When did the symptoms start? _____

● Is there any:

    Pain?

        ● Sharp?

        ● Dull?

        ● In one body location, or many locations?

_____

        ● Constant or now and then? Any pattern?

_____

    Vomiting?

        ● How often? Any pattern? _____

_____

Headache? _____

Fever?

    ● How high? _____

    ● When did you last take your child's
temperature? _____

Swelling? If so, where? _____

Bleeding? _____

Discharge? _____

Bulging in the groin, abdomen, or scrotum? _____

Skin discoloration or rash? _____

● Any changes in:

    ● Urination? _____

    ● Bowel movements? _____

    ● Appetite? _____

● Any difficulties breathing or swallowing? _____

● Can the child's limbs be moved without pain? _____

● Any other symptoms the doctor/health-care professional should
know about? _____

_____

● What medications, if any, is the child taking? _____

_____

    ● Any allergies to medications? _____

_____

● Has this ever happened before? If so, when? _____

_____

● Does anything offer relief? _____

Introduction

Parents are always deeply concerned when a child develops signs and symptoms of a potentially serious medical problem. What's wrong? What can it mean? Should I take the child to the doctor right away? *Childhood Symptoms* attempts to anticipate the types of questions a parent might like to ask the child's doctor and then provides clear answers to those questions.

Since its first edition in 1985, *Childhood Symptoms* has been completely revised and updated. The basic goal of the book is to explain to parents and other concerned adults the significance of virtually all the signs and symptoms of diseases, disorders, and developmental problems that can affect infants, children, and adolescents. Entries are presented in alphabetical order in two sections: "Diseases, Disorders, and Conditions" and "Complaints, Concerns, and Problems." In addition, an extensive system of cross-references, indicated by a term in SMALL CAPITAL LETTERS within the text of an entry or at the end of an entry, helps direct the reader from a specific symptom to those conditions in which that symptom may be important diagnostic evidence for the physician. The reader obtains a fully integrated discussion of specific symptoms and their most likely underlying cause.

In most cases a group of signs and symptoms will emerge that forms a pattern of a suspected illness. Only a qualified physician, with proper experience in identifying such patterns, can diagnose a suspected problem and offer the most effective modern treatment. A doctor often has to study the results of specific laboratory tests and other diagnostic procedures before confirming the diagnosis.

Readers must realize that the information contained in *Childhood*

Symptoms should never be used as a substitute for professional medical care or used to self-diagnose any specific problem a child may have. Rather, it is designed to provide helpful and general information that can be discussed openly with a child's physician. A parent or any daily caretaker who is knowledgeable about the signs and symptoms of childhood diseases is in a better position to aid the doctor in the main goal of returning an ill child to health as soon as possible.

DISEASES, DISORDERS, AND CONDITIONS

A

Acne

Acne vulgaris — the Latin name for common acne — involves an in-flammation of the sebaceous (oil-secreting) glands that produces pimples, the small red swellings that often exude pus. Acne usually appears on the face as well as the chest and back.

Although acne sometimes afflicts preteenagers and adults, this skin disorder is most common during adolescence. This is the time that androgenic hormones are first secreted into the bloodstream. Unfortunately, it is also the time at which most young people take a new and sudden interest in how they look and whether they are attractive.

Androgenic hormones cause increased activity of the sebaceous glands of the skin. Sebum, the sticky substance produced by these glands, sometimes fills and stretches the skin pores. The result: black-heads. These blackheads block the pores, preventing natural skin oils from reaching the surface. As these blocked oils collect beneath the outside surface of the skin, they form tiny cysts. When the cysts break, harmful bacteria can cross the skin's "protective barrier," causing inflammation and infection.

As affected adolescents know, there is acne and there is *acne*. The so-called Pillsbury Classifications cover four degrees of severity:

- Grade I is a relatively mild condition in which there are blackheads and whiteheads and a vaguely pimply appearance, but no serious interference with the adolescent's appearance — except possibly in his or her own estimation.
- Grade II features more and more enlarged whiteheads that are deeply impacted and may cover the whole face.
- In Grade III there are enlarged and swollen, pus-filled eruptions in addition to blackheads and whiteheads.
- In Grade IV acne the sufferer's face is likely to be covered with large

3

raw-looking, purple-colored cysts in addition to the smaller lesions. This is truly disfiguring and deeply traumatic to the affected teenager.

There is no good time to have acne. Well-meaning parents — and even well-meaning doctors — can reassure adolescents all they want that having acne is part of growing up and that it will not last forever. Adolescents know better. The fact of the matter is that except for the mildest Grade I acne, the lesions *are* unsightly and disfiguring, and to an adolescent — whose wait for the next school dance seems like forever — the thought of waiting two, four, or six years for this condition to clear is intolerable.

ACTION — Treatment depends on severity. Regardless of the grade of acne, the pimples that form around pore openings should not be squeezed; this may spread any infection that is present or cause a second infection from harmful bacteria on the skin surface or underneath fingernails. Since it is seldom an easy task for sufferers or their parents to determine if both inflammation and infection are present, it is best to consult a doctor or perhaps a dermatologist (a skin specialist), who is apt to be aware of the newest acne treatments, such as isotretinoin, available under the trade name Accutane, a prescription drug that can be taken for extremely severe cystic acne. Though an excellent treatment, there are potentially some very serious side effects, most notably the effects on the unborn fetus if the user is pregnant.

In simple cases, it may be sufficient simply to wash the affected areas with soap and water and apply drying solutions. Antibacterial soaps seem to offer no added benefit. Several nonprescription products may help. Among the most useful are those that contain benzoyl peroxide, a chemical that helps dry the skin and remove excess oil. But use of these products should be discontinued at the first sign of excessive itching, burning, redness, or extreme drying of the skin.

Adenoids

See TONSILLITIS

AIDS

Acquired immune deficiency syndrome — a disease caused by the fluid-carried human immuno-deficiency virus (HIV), which attacks the body's immune system, leaving the body unable to defend itself against infections, pneumonia, and certain cancers.

AIDS has been called the modern plague, and so it seems. From the time it was first recognized in the United States in 1981, it has been an insidious disease — it can incubate and reside in the body without producing symptoms for as long as a decade, then wipe out a life in a matter of months, or years at most. Even when AIDS is unsuspected but present in a person, it is alive and able to be transmitted unwittingly to the innocent or the careless.

As much as we would like to hope otherwise, children get AIDS too. They can get it while in the womb or during birth from an infected mother. The prognosis for such children is very poor, and most live very short, unhappy lives. Children also get AIDS in the same ways adults do:

- Via the exchange of bodily fluids during "unsafe" homosexual, bisexual, and heterosexual activity
- From blood transfusions and from receiving blood products if one is a hemophiliac (although since 1985, blood tests have reduced this mode of AIDS transmission to near zero)
- By sharing needles with infected intravenous drug users

Children can also get AIDS if they are sexually abused by someone with the disease.

AIDS symptoms include enlarged, painful lymph nodes in the neck or armpits, unexplained weight loss, a dry cough, purple bumps under the skin, night sweats, chills, fatigue, and diarrhea.

People die not from AIDS, but from diseases that overcome the body once its immune system is too ravaged by AIDS to fight back. Certain cancers, such as Kaposi's sarcoma, and pneumocystic carinii pneumonia and other opportunistic infections are the usual causes of death. AIDS also affects the brain and can lead to slow dementia and death.

These are the horrors. What needs to be done to protect children is, first, to educate them about the causes and conditions under which AIDS can be transmitted. Safe sex — that is, with the use of a condom — is to be strongly encouraged in sexually active youths. Intravenous drug use needs to be discouraged at all costs.

It is a balancing act, because there is a need, especially among younger children, to alert them to the dangers without creating nightmarish fears and phobias that lead them to think that AIDS is lurking around every corner. It is important to relay to children that AIDS can be transmitted only in the very few ways mentioned above; it is not spread by coughing or sneezing, by eating from utensils or dishes in restaurants, by swimming in public pools or using public toilets, or during any casual contact. Being around someone with AIDS — perhaps a classmate — poses no danger either.

ACTION — There is no cure for AIDS. There is no vaccine to prevent it, and there are only a few expensive drugs, such as AZT (offered in the form of a fruit-flavored syrup), that seem to slow it down; the drug DDI, particularly, has been shown in studies to sharply reduce levels of the AIDS virus in children. However, use of these or other similar drugs carries some potentially serious side effects.

More information about AIDS can be obtained by calling the 24-hour AIDS Information Hot Line of the Public Health Service: 800-342-AIDS (202-245-6887 in Alaska and Hawaii; call collect); 800-344-SIDA is a Spanish-language hot line.

Allergic Rhinitis

See HAY FEVER

Allergy

Any condition in which a person becomes unusually sensitive to some substance(s) or physical agent(s).

With allergies, nothing happens during the first encounter between the child and the substance or agent. In fact, it may take several years for an individual to become "sensitized" to the point at which an allergy develops. But once this sensitization occurs, the now-allergic person suffers a typical reaction every time he or she encounters the offending material.

The substance that triggers an allergic reaction in a sensitized person is called an *allergen.* It may be pollen, animal hair or dander, fur, house dust, an insect bite or sting, certain foods, some antibiotics (especially penicillin), or many other things. An allergic reaction may also be caused or heightened by emotional states or by cold, heat, and sunlight. Most allergies are more annoying than serious, although in rare instances a severe allergic reaction called ANAPHYLACTIC SHOCK can be a direct threat to life.

Children as well as adults are subject to a wide variety of allergies. Sometimes allergies have a hereditary basis, although a specific allergy is not always passed on to children. Recent studies have linked allergic reactions and ASTHMA to certain foods eaten by the pregnant mother that are passed on to and sensitize the baby in the womb; later, when the child comes in contact with these allergens again — either in solid food or from the mother's milk during breast-feeding — allergic reactions can occur. Smoking by the pregnant mother has also been implicated in making the unborn child more susceptible to respiratory infections.

The most common sites for allergic reaction are the skin, the air passages to the lungs, the nose, and the digestive tract. Disorders include ECZEMA, HIVES, allergic BRONCHITIS, ASTHMA, HAY FEVER, and some conditions affecting the intestinal tract.

An allergic reaction involves the breakdown of the immune mechanisms, the body's normal defense against disease. The body normally responds to bacterial and viral infections by producing protective substances called *antibodies*, which are released into the bloodstream to attack the bacteria or virus. In many cases, the protective substances remain in the body for years, providing partial or total immunity to further attacks of the same disease. The body of an allergic person treats certain substances — for example, pollen, feathers, or shellfish — as if they were disease-causing invaders such as bacteria. The basic mechanism of the allergic reaction is the same; it is the site that is affected that determines the specific outcome. For example, allergens that meet allergic antibodies in the skin cause hives.

Histamine plays a special role in allergies. Histamine is a normal body substance concentrated largely in those tissues that have direct or indirect contact with the air: the skin, the lining of the nose, and the lungs. In the case of injury or infection, certain amounts of histamine are normally released into affected tissues. Histamine causes a dilation, or opening, of the smaller blood vessels at the site of an injury and contributes to the so-called inflammatory response, which is a natural feature of the healing process. This response allows the escape of some *plasma* (the clear fluid portion of the blood) through the walls of tiny blood vessels and into surrounding tissues, which results in the swelling that accompanies many injuries and infections.

Often it is the sudden release of histamine that is responsible for the signs and symptoms of an allergic reaction. In a sensitized individual, when an invading allergen comes in contact with a body cell to which an allergic antibody is attached, it causes the dramatic response known as the allergic reaction. Histamine is released from such cells in greater amounts than would be normal; that is, normal in the case of injury or infection. Depending on the site of the allergic reaction, this can cause swelling, redness, and itching of the skin, sometimes with the formation of wheals or bumps; inflammation and swelling of the mucous membranes of the nose, causing nasal congestion or a stuffy nose; constriction or spasm of the *bronchioles*, the small air passages in the lungs; and increased activity of the digestive tract.

ACTION — Relief can frequently be obtained by taking antihistamines — "anti" meaning that they act to neutralize or inhibit the action of histamine. For relatively minor problems, sufferers may use an antihistamine that is available without prescription. More powerful antihistamines for more severe allergic reactions can be prescribed by a physician. Since the age of the child and the exact nature of the allergy are important factors to consider, parents may want to check with the child's doctor and also carefully read the children's dose information accompanying any nonprescription preparation.

Prevention, however, is the best course: Parents should do everything possible to keep allergic children away from the obvious allergens. Dust is difficult to avoid, but certain foods are not, and neither are animals to which the child reacts. Children may love to have dogs or cats in the house, but if having the animals causes allergy attacks or much discomfort, it is a relationship that needs to be discontinued, at least for the time being.

Amebic Dysentery

A disease of the intestinal tract caused by the infectious single-cell organisms called Endamoeba histolytica.

Symptoms of amebic dysentery caused by inflammation of the mucous membranes of the intestine include abdominal pain and severe diarrhea with blood or mucus typically being passed in loose, watery stools. The disease occurs worldwide, but is more common in tropical countries or underdeveloped areas where standards of hygiene are inadequate.

The disease is spread from human feces or stools that contain a cystic form of the ameba. In this form, the ameba cells build a protective wall around themselves. If they are swallowed in food or water that is contaminated with them, they eventually shed this wall in the human intestines, where they begin to multiply and cause dysentery.

At first the inflammation of the walls of the colon (large intestine) causes the child to experience painful passage of stools, which are often stained with mucus and blood. The infection may cause erosion or ulceration of the intestinal wall, leading to abscesses.

For diagnostic purposes, microscopic examination must be made of the child's stool. It is especially important for the doctor to distinguish the disease from BACILLARY DYSENTERY.

ACTION — Treatment depends on severity. Bed rest and a bland diet are necessary until all signs of infection have disappeared. In many cases drugs such as emetine or metronidazole may be prescribed. It is important to obtain appropriate medical care because, if left untreated, the infection can enter the bloodstream and be carried to the liver, lungs, or, more rarely, to the pericardium (the sac that surrounds the heart).

Anal Fissure

A tear or cracking of the lining around the anus (the external opening at the end of the digestive tract).

The tear usually results from the child having a large hard bowel movement or straining excessively when going to the bathroom. On occasion it may occur after bouts of diarrhea, when unusually runny stools have irritated the area.

Generally speaking, the condition should be suspected when blood, usually bright red in color, is noted on the outside of the bowel movement or, in toilet-trained youngsters, on toilet paper used for wiping. The amount of blood is usually small — less than a teaspoon — and bleeding generally stops spontaneously. If the bleeding is larger in volume or if the blood is mixed with the bowel movement, there may be a problem higher in the intestine. Medical attention should be sought at once.

A parent can usually determine if an anal fissure is present. If the child's or infant's buttocks are spread wide enough, the fissure will appear as a raw-looking crack around the rim of the anal opening itself, with normal tissue on either side.

ACTION — Treatment can be both direct and indirect — usually a combination works best. The fissure itself should be thoroughly cleansed with mild soap and water after each bowel movement. Sitz baths are especially useful. The older child can soak his or her bottom in slightly warm, but not hot, water for 20 minutes two or three times a day. The infant or toddler who needs support must be held so that the water soaks the anal area. At times, special creams may be helpful, but parents should first discuss this with the child's physician. Inserting glycerin suppositories lubricates the area and eases passage of stools in children who are straining.

When hard bowel movements seem to be causing the difficulty, a change in diet may help, since more roughage is needed. Bran cereals or commercially available stool softeners hold more water in the stool, making it softer and easier to pass. Infants may benefit from the addition of a stool softener to a bottle of milk, formula, or water. If the problem persists, a physician should be consulted.

Anaphylactic Shock

The most serious, potentially lethal form of allergic reaction.

In anaphylactic shock, also known as anaphylactic reaction, the sensitized person experiences a sudden and explosive reaction when confronted by the allergen. Anaphylactic shock may be caused by injection of a drug such as penicillin, use of a diagnostic agent such as x-ray contrast medium, the sting of a bee or wasp, or eating some seemingly innocuous food such as strawberries or shellfish. A typical reaction includes severe interference with breathing (caused by spasm of the tiny air passages in the lungs or swelling of the throat); hypotension (a sudden drop in blood pressure); and, on some occasions, convulsions and loss of consciousness. In rare instances death can occur. Anaphylactic reactions are life threatening but not necessarily fatal. But to the child suddenly stricken by difficult breathing and the cold, clammy kind of faintness that accompanies a sudden drop in blood pressure, the distinction is very fine indeed.

ACTION — Emergency treatment of anaphylactic shock includes injection of epinephrine (adrenaline) and administration of an antihistamine (either by injection or, if the child is able to swallow, by mouth). Sometimes it may also be necessary to add to blood volume by intravenously administering a special salt solution.

It is helpful to have some tablet-form antihistamines on hand for emergency use. Large doses of over-the-counter ones may do the trick, or your child's pediatrician may prescribe a stronger antihistamine. A kit containing epinephrine and a chewable antihistamine is available by prescription and should *always* be kept on hand if you have a child who has a history of severe reactions. Parents can also discuss desensitization with the child's doctor if the child has a history of severe reactions to bee stings and other allergens.

Regardless of the availability of emergency medical treatment, the best precaution is avoiding any substance to which the child is known to be sensitive. In the case of wasps and bees, sensitive children should stay away from areas where they are known to nest and flourish. They should avoid wearing bright or pastel-color clothing when outdoors, and parents should consider avoiding colognes or scented lotions that could attract insects.

See also ALLERGY, STINGS

Anemia

A condition in which the red blood cells are reduced below a certain volume or do not have adequate oxygen-carrying capacity.

There are many causes for anemia. In nutritional anemia, the most common form, there is simply not enough iron available for blood-cell formation. Sometimes infants who consume large quantities of milk and very little else show this kind of anemia. Loss of blood, for whatever reason, may be a cause, as can some infections and certain chronic illnesses. There are also congenital (present-at-birth) or familial anemias, such as SICKLE-CELL DISEASE, which result from defective formation of red blood cells.

Children who are anemic appear pale, listless, and inattentive. A severely anemic child tires easily or perhaps becomes short of breath when active. Excessive thirst may be a problem, and adolescents sometimes chew or suck on ice cubes. However, it is frequently the case that no significant symptoms or signs are noted by parents, and only blood tests show the anemia.

Iron deficiency may lead to a behavior called *pica*, which is a craving for eating unnatural, abnormal items, such as dirt. The danger of pica is that, depending on the bizarre substance eaten, it could result in lead or other poisoning.

ACTION — Both the diagnosis and the treatment of an anemic condition should be carried out by a qualified physician. Sometimes a blood specialist, called a hematologist, is consulted. If a child is listless, parents should not attempt to treat the condition by giving iron supplements. First of all, if the child is not really anemic, the iron is of no value. Second, and more important, large amounts of iron can be dangerous to children. Too much iron can cause gastrointestinal upset, staining of teeth, and, if really excessive, *siderosis* (a disease that results from excess iron circulating in the blood).

See BLOOD in Appendix I: Norms and Values

Anorexia Nervosa

An abnormal and prolonged suppression of appetite related to mental or emotional illness and characterized by excessive weight loss, often resulting in an emaciated, almost skeletal appearance.

The condition primarily affects preadolescent and adolescent girls and seems to be connected with body image and an irrational fear of being overweight. The condition is not associated with any underlying physical disease initially.

Although these individuals frequently seem never to eat, they do not always lose their appetites altogether. Indeed, many girls alternate anorexia nervosa with periods of BULIMIA, an excessively abnormal increase in appetite. They may go on eating binges and consume huge quantities of their favorite foods, such as chocolate sundaes, before they then force themselves to vomit. A poll of *Seventeen* magazine readers found that 2 percent of girls are anorexic, while somewhere between 5 percent and 20 percent of girls are bulimic.

Preoccupation with food often leads anorexics to collect diets and recipes, prepare large and fancy dinners for other people, and sometimes hoard and waste food.

Emotionally, they are often quite depressed. Behaviorally, they often become highly manipulative, managing to get what they want out of concerned family members or professionals by using eating as a bargaining tool.

Physically, the child with anorexia nervosa may show abnormal patterns of growth in body and facial hair, low blood pressure, low body temperature, and menstrual difficulties, including amenorrhea (having no menstrual periods). In fact, one theory is that some girls fall prey to anorexia nervosa because they are unsure of and frightened about growing up and maturing sexually, and anorexic behavior can stunt sexual development.

Underlying causes seem to be multiple and complicated, and recovery can be slow. Therefore, the advice "the sooner the better" applies when it comes to treatment; otherwise, the disorder can lead to severe nutritional deficiencies and even death by starvation or related complications.

ACTION — Medical treatment must be sought. When there has been significant weight loss, hospitalization may be required, initially with the possibility of tube or "forced" feeding. A useful psychotherapeutic approach seems to be allowing the patient to regress to more and more infantile states but using a firm approach when it comes to feeding. Gradually, independence and more mature behavior are encouraged.

Family therapy with a counselor skilled in dealing with anorexia nervosa patients and their parents may be advisable.

More information concerning anorexia nervosa and other eating disorders may be obtained by calling the following toll-free numbers: Bulimia-Anorexia Self-Help, 800-762-3334; Mercy Hospital Eating Disorder Unit, 800-332-2832.

See BULIMIA

Appendicitis

An inflammation of the appendix, a small wormlike tube, closed at its free end, that juts down from the cecum, a kind of pouch that forms the beginning portion of the large intestine.

The appendix is about the length and half the diameter of an adult's little finger, and it usually hangs freely within the abdominal cavity. The interior of the appendix is very narrow. Sometimes hard pieces of waste matter or foreign bodies become trapped within it, causing an obstruction leading to severe inflammation. It can also become inflamed as the result of a general infection or when an abscess spreads from a nearby area.

Children of any age can be stricken with appendicitis, although adolescents seem to be at greater risk. It has been estimated that in the United States 4 out of every 1,000 children undergo appendectomies each year. For unknown reasons, the peak incidence of appendicitis occurs in autumn and spring, and males are affected more often than females.

Symptoms and signs vary from one individual to the next. Usually pain begins in the middle of the abdomen or the pit of the stomach and later moves to the lower right side of the abdomen. Nausea and vomiting generally develop early on. Because the peritoneum (the membrane that lines the abdominal cavity) is irritated, movement causes pain; coughing hurts, and a child may walk bent over. If the appendix has ruptured, a child's temperature may reach 104°F (40°C). Recently, ultrasound has been used successfully to better diagnose acute appendicitis in children.

In an acute attack of appendicitis, the blood supply to the appendix is interrupted. This, in turn, can lead to gangrene, that is, death of part of its tissues. If the infected appendix ruptures, PERITONITIS may develop.

ACTION — Treatment of acute appendicitis involves surgical removal of the inflamed appendix. It is a relatively simple operation that requires only a short stay in the hospital. If the slightest suspicion exists that the child's tummy ache could be appendicitis, *never* give a laxative. This could hasten rupture. The first rule is: Call a physician at the very first hint that the child may have appendicitis. Delay could also result in a rupture, which can be life threatening, even in today's era of powerful antibiotics.

Arthritis

A disease of the bony joints in which there is both swelling and pain.

Occasionally, arthritis is a localized or isolated problem that may stem from infection by invading bacteria. However, most commonly the swelling and pain occur because of some systemic disease such as JUVENILE RHEUMATOID ARTHRITIS, RHEUMATIC FEVER (the most common cause of arthritis in children), or LUPUS ERYTHEMATOSUS.

ACTION — Parents should not give their child aspirin or some other anti-inflammatory over-the-counter medication in order to mask the symptoms, hoping the problem is temporary and will pass. Especially since serious diseases may be involved, the first indication of swollen, painful joints requires an immediate visit to a physician, followed possibly by consultation with a specialist.

Ascariasis

Infestation of the intestines with a specific type of parasitic round-worm called Ascaris lumbricoides.

Children under the age of about 12 years are most likely to be affected by ascariasis, and the possible complication of INTESTINAL OBSTRUCTION is noted mostly in children under the age of 6.

The eggs of these worms develop in soil. Very young children may take them in simply by putting dirt into their mouths. Older children may become infected as a result of putting contaminated fingers or toys into their mouths. The eggs hatch inside the intestines and then may be circulated to the lungs and the epiglottis (a lidlike structure that covers the larynx or voice box). Here they may be reswallowed and go back to the intestines as adult worms, so more eggs are laid and the cycle continues.

Often the child shows no symptoms and the condition goes unnoticed unless a parent happens to find a worm in the child's bowel movement. If symptoms do occur, children usually show intermittent pain in the abdomen or in the pit of the stomach; loss of appetite and perhaps some weight loss; and, if the worms pass through the lungs, a kind of PNEUMONIA or perhaps ASTHMA-like episodes.

Diagnosis is made by identifying a worm that is passed in the child's stools or by finding eggs in a stool sample and examining them under a microscope.

ACTION — Treatment typically involves the use of antiparasitic drugs such as piperazine citrate, pyrantel pamoate, or mebendazole.

Asthma

A disorder that affects the small air passages of the lungs, constricting them so that breathing becomes difficult and very labored. Typically, there are sudden attacks of breathlessness and wheezing, and a bout leaves the sufferer exhausted.

Many factors can cause or contribute to asthma, which afflicts nearly 10 million Americans, including between 4 percent and 8 percent of U.S. youngsters. Asthma is the leading chronic disease of childhood and the leading cause of medically related school absences. Three major factors are ALLERGY (including a family history of allergies such as HAY FEVER, ECZEMA, and asthma itself), emotional stress, and infection (perhaps due to damage caused to the respiratory tract, which makes the airway sensitive). Asthma can start at any age, but when it begins early in childhood, it is most commonly caused by an allergy; however, the incidence of infection-caused asthma seems to be on the rise, especially in children hospitalized with respiratory syncytial virus BRONCHIOLITIS. It has been noted, though, that such children may outgrow their asthma earlier than those with allergic asthma.

Inhaled pollen, dust (and house-dust mites), molds, and animal danders as well as certain foods are common offenders. When the foreign substance causes a sudden release of histamine from the cells of tissues in the lungs' smaller air passages, mucous membranes swell and the muscles tighten, causing the constriction. In addition, thick and sticky mucus is secreted, further blocking air passages and making breathing even more difficult. In order to get enough air, affected children may have to sit upright and forcibly lift and drop their shoulders.

Allergic asthma can be seasonal (for example, a reaction to high pollen count) or it may occur at any time of the year. In most cases, asthmatic attacks occur in isolated episodes, although they can last from a few minutes or hours to up to several days in chronic patients. In severe cases, asthmatic attacks can be extremely frightening to both the children and their parents. The victim often believes that suffocation is taking place, and this fear only serves to intensify the attack. Therefore, it is essential that concerned parents shield their own anxiety from the child as much as possible — there is enough dread already. Asthma can account for deaths, but the figure is very small — less than 1 per 100,000 in the 5- to 14-year-old age group.

Even in the presence of a known allergen (the substance that triggers an allergic reaction), the emotional factor may be more obvious in children than in adults. In children susceptible to asthma, tension at home or constant parental arguing can play a key role in the frequency and severity of attacks.

Both parents and an asthmatic child can take some reassurance from the fact that children often — but not always — outgrow their asthma, although sometimes it is replaced in later years by some other allergic condition, such as HAY FEVER. In some chronic sufferers, the outlook is not so promising, and a doctor should be consulted at regular intervals for the monitoring and treatment of the disorder.

Parents need have few worries about the effect of athletic activity on asthmatic children. Although it was once thought that sports activity was detrimental to the child's health, recent studies have shown that it may actually be beneficial. There is such a thing as exercise-induced asthma, but it is not serious; in fact, several U.S. Olympic athletes have won medals despite their asthma. So long as the child uses a bronchodilator (see below) 20 to 30 minutes before the activity, he or she should be fine for hours.

ACTION — Asthmatic attacks often occur at night. When a bout starts, try to stay as calm as possible. Sit near the child or on the edge of the bed and speak softly and reassuringly during the attack and for a short time afterward. However, be careful not to overdo, as too much attention and concern over a long period can be as bad as panic in adding to the child's nervousness about an asthmatic bout.

Various drugs exist that can be prescribed by the child's physician to lessen the frequency and severity of the attacks. The doctor can also help by suggesting ways to alleviate tensions or family problems that may be contributing to the asthma.

Bronchodilators (medicines that dilate the bronchial tubes) and some antiasthmatic drugs are available without a doctor's prescription. However, these over-the-counter products should *never* be used unless a physician has actually made the diagnosis of asthma. Also, if such products seem to cause a worsening of the child's condition, medical help should be sought at once.

The National Jewish Center for Immunology and Respiratory Medicine operates a 24-hour telephone service offering free information about asthma. It is called the Lung Line and can be reached by dialing 800-222-LUNG (303-355-5864 in Colorado). The National Allergy and Asthma Network offers a similar service and can be reached by dialing 800-878-4403.

Athlete's Foot

A fungus infection of the foot, characterized by redness, itching, cracking, and scaling of the skin, especially between the toes, and sometimes by the formation of watery blisters.

This condition is not common in young children, but it may become a recurring problem for preadolescent and adolescent youths who engage in sports programs or are otherwise in settings where showers and other facilities are shared by many pairs of youthful bare feet, such as at summer camp.

Children's feet often sweat excessively, and the moisture may cause irritation. Also, allergic reactions to dyes and glues used in footwear may cause symptoms similar to those of athlete's foot. Microscopic examination of a scraping from the skin settles the question of diagnosis.

ACTION — Managing the disease requires some close attention to the frequent washing of clothes, bed linens, and towels. Children should be instructed to be sure to dry between their toes after bathing, and they should avoid footwear that prevents an adequate amount of air from reaching the feet. Mild infections can be treated by dusting the feet with an absorbent antifungal powder such as zinc undecylenate. In more persistent infections, a physician may prescribe application of clotrimazole or miconazole nitrate.

Attention-Deficit Disorders

Conditions caused by some neurological imbalance, contributing to the child's difficulty in maintaining alertness or attention to some task at hand. Children may also experience problems with impulsivity and HYPERACTIVE BEHAVIOR.

Formerly tagged as having minimal brain dysfunction (MBD), children or adolescents with attention-deficit disorders (ADDs) or attention-deficit hyperactivity disorders (ADHDs) generally have perfectly normal or even above-normal intelligence. About one third of children with ADDs will have the condition to some degree when they become adults. Some experts suggest that this condition is hereditary and that when a child exhibits ADD behavior, it is not surprising to discover that the parent has the disorder to some extent and may not even be aware of it.

Current medical thinking is that ADDs are biological, not psychological, in nature, and that proper medication (usually methylphenidate) may help children deal with society at large (and with themselves) as well as compete academically. In conjunction with the medication — which seems, in many cases, to do wonders — counseling is valuable in helping the child deal with the anxiety, anger, embarrassment, and frustration his or her condition may cause; many of these children desperately want to be and try to be still and attentive but cannot impose any control over themselves without medication.

Some doctors, though believing in the medical nature of ADDs, believe that psychoactive drugs should be used only as a last resort in extreme cases and that other techniques — such as dietary modifications or relaxation therapies — should be given a first chance to effect changes in the child's behavior. They make the case that the hyperactivity or lack of attention that typifies ADDs is merely in the eye of the beholder; that is, a very active child in a quiet setting may be thought to have an ADD, while that same child in a more active setting may be indistinguishable from the other normally rambunctious children. They also suggest that what is thought to be ADD might simply be a nonmedical discipline or behavior problem.

Dietary changes seem, in some cases, to improve the condition. Some parents attest to the fact that elimination of certain foods, such as wheat and dairy products, produce noticeable, even remarkable changes. The so-called Feingold diet to fight hyperactivity requires children to refrain from eating any foods with artificial colorings, flavorings, and preservatives in them, as well as staying away from certain chemicals prevalent in the household environment.

ACTION — The combined efforts of parents, medical and psychological professionals, and the child's teachers are necessary to deal with this condition. Parents who suspect an attention-deficit disorder in their child should promptly seek professional assessment.

Autism

A severe disorder of communication and behavior, sometimes called infantile autism or infantile psychosis, characterized by a profound and almost total withdrawal from all human contact — even an avoidance of eye contact.

The cause of infantile autism is unknown. There is no evidence to suggest that the condition is associated with parental rejection, as was once believed. It is typically noted during a child's first few months of life and invariably is present by the time the child reaches the age of 3 years. It affects approximately 4 children per 100,000 and is 4 times as common in boys as in girls.

Autistic children repel attempts at cuddling or play and they may engage in bizarre activities such as banging their heads against walls.

They often form attachments to inanimate objects and show an obsessive need for sameness or ritual. If their routines are disrupted, they may throw violent TEMPER TANTRUMS. There is often considerable MENTAL RETARDATION, but even when this is not the case, the development of speech is seriously delayed or virtually absent.

If communicative speech does not develop by about the age of 5, the outlook is generally poor. Psychological tests are difficult to administer but, in skillful hands, can help define the limits of expected development. If the child's general intelligence is not severely impaired, a normal school education may be possible for those children who are amenable to behavior-therapy techniques and whose parents are patient enough to apply them after professional guidance.

A recent study strongly indicates that certain kinds of autism are inherited, and that if parents have one autistic child, the risk of having another with this condition is slightly less than 20 percent; if there are two autistic children, the chance of a third being autistic is more than 35 percent. Genetic and other counseling for such parents is strongly advised.

ACTION — Generally speaking, no specific treatment exists, although tranquilizers are sometimes prescribed to relieve symptoms such as screaming attacks and extreme hyperactivity. In severe forms of autism it may be necessary to institutionalize the child.

B

Bacillary Dysentery

An acute infectious disease, also known as shigellosis, *of the large intestine caused by a particular type of bacteria called* Shigella.

The microorganisms that cause bacillary dysentery are transmitted in the stools of infected persons and may be picked up and carried by flies or through the handling of contaminated foods or other objects. The disease is most common in areas of overcrowding, where sanitation is poor.

The sufferer typically experiences a profuse diarrhea in which the frequent stools are watery and streaked with mucus and blood. Other symptoms and signs include abdominal cramps, spasmodic contractions of the muscle ring that surrounds the anus, general weakness, and fever. Children with bacillary dysentery may run extremely high fevers and experience convulsions. Diagnosis is made by identifying the bacteria in a stool sample. Often an examination of the bottommost section of the large intestine shows certain destructive changes in the intestinal wall that rarely occur in AMEBIC DYSENTERY.

The incubation period from infection to symptoms is usually two to three days. The severity of the disease depends on the exact species of bacteria and the sufferer's general health. If a child is suffering from malnutrition or is already run down because of another disease, the death rate can be high. However, in the majority of uncomplicated cases, the disease runs its course and spontaneously clears up in about a week. More severe infections may last for six weeks or more.

ACTION — Bed rest and fluid replacement, administered either by mouth or through a vein, constitute the best therapeutic approach. Fluid replacement is necessary because the infection causes serious loss of essential body fluids and the elements they contain, particularly salt. In more severe cases, a physician may want to prescribe antibiotics.

Bacterial Infections

Invasion of the organs or tissues of the body by one or more types of pathogenic (disease-causing) bacteria.

Bacteria are single-celled microorganisms so small that over a million can exist on the head of a pin. They are classified in three ways:

1. General shape: coccus (round), bacillus (rodlike), and spirillum (spiral)
2. Whether they retain a gram stain (a special laboratory dye), a classification method that helps indicate which of various antibiotics are appropriate to treat the specific bacteria
3. Whether the microorganism is aerobic (requires oxygen in order to live) or anaerobic (able to survive without oxygen)

Bacteria exist naturally in soil, in fresh water, and in the sea. They live in the mouth, in the digestive tract, and on the skin — usually without causing any problem. But sometimes they get misplaced and cause trouble. For example, some types of bacteria that are harmless in the intestines can cause considerable irritation in a girl's vagina if careless wiping sweeps the bacteria to the area.

In a suitable environment, such as an open wound, a small number of bacteria can multiply into several million within a relatively short time. The microorganisms generally reproduce by splitting into two identical cells. Some of them are able to form a thick wall around themselves, becoming a cyst or spore that is resistant to heat, drying, or the effects of chemicals intended to kill them.

Most bacterial infections can be treated successfully with one or more of the antibiotic drugs. An antibiotic is a chemical substance produced by certain species of bacteria, molds, or other microorganisms. When it comes in contact with other species of germs, it can kill them or inhibit their growth and multiplication. Antibiotics are among the few drugs that can cure a disease by removing its cause. Penicillin was one of the first of the modern antibiotics to be discovered, and it is still considered to be one of the most useful in treating a wide range of infections. Today, however, physicians have many different antibiotics to choose from in the treatment of specific bacterial infections.

Not all antibiotics act in the same way, nor are they equally effective against a specific bacterial infection. The one that is prescribed by the child's physician depends on the nature and severity of the infection, whether the child is especially sensitive to the drug (for example, some people are extremely sensitive or allergic to penicillin and may experience ANAPHYLACTIC SHOCK if it is given), and whether the bacteria may have become resistant to a particular antibiotic.

ACTION — It is very important to see that the child completes the full course of antibiotic therapy exactly as the physician directs. That is, if the doctor says the child should take the drug for ten days, it should not be stopped two or three days after the first dose just because the child seems to look and feel better. Taking too little of the drug or failing to take it at the proper intervals can allow the infection to progress and may also cause an immune effect in the bacteria, so that the antibiotic will not work. This occurs because natural selection allows the stronger microorganisms to predominate so that treatment-resistant strains emerge.

It is also important that the child not be given more of the drug than is prescribed and that doses not be given more frequently than instructed. Either of these overloads may result in annoying or even potentially dangerous side effects. If nothing else, it is costly and ineffective. If treatment is to be effective, the physician's instructions must be followed to the letter. Otherwise, recovery time may be greatly prolonged or complications may develop.

Compare VIRAL INFECTIONS

Bee Stings

See STINGS

Birth Injuries

Any injury that occurs just before or during the time of an infant's delivery.

Some studies suggest that birth injuries may happen in as many as 7 out of every 1,000 births. Most of them occur even with the most expert obstetrical care and are considered unavoidable.

Most babies emerge headfirst. Not uncommonly, especially if the infant is large, the collarbone or clavicle may be fractured during the process. Newborns with fractured collarbones tend not to use the arm on the affected side, or they may cry when the arm is moved. Sometimes swelling and a bluish discoloration are noticed in the skin that lies over the collarbone area. This injury is not a serious one, and the fracture usually heals within two or three weeks. Fractures of other bones may occur and are usually noticed shortly after birth. Treatment is undertaken by the medical team attending the birth.

Sometimes when a considerable amount of traction has been required to get the baby out in a hurry, nerves coming from the spinal cord or in an extremity may be injured, in which case parents may notice that the baby does not use the affected limb normally. Recovery of nerve function depends on whether the nerves were torn or just stretched.

By far the most common site of injury is the head. The infant's head sustains a considerable amount of pressure as the mother's uterine contractions push the baby through the cervix and down the birth canal. The scalp may be swollen and discolored in places, and the skull may appear elongated or pointy. This condition is called *molding*, and it usually clears up within a few weeks. However, on rare occasions the head injury may be severe enough to cause a skull fracture or bleeding into the brain. Should this happen, the baby quickly develops symptoms that alert the nurses and doctors to start therapy. The nature of that therapy depends on the degree of involvement, but modern techniques of treating tiny infants have substantially lowered the rates of death or serious impairment.

Rather frequently, a localized area of bleeding occurs on a baby's skull; it looks like a large bump or goose egg. The congested blood that causes these bumps is usually absorbed by the baby's body in two to three weeks. On occasion the lump may last longer. No treatment is required, and parents need not be concerned.

Sometimes a small bright red area of bleeding shows in the white of a newborn baby's eyes because of pressures that occur on the head during normal birth processes. This too should cause no parental concern. It clears up by itself.

Similarly, parents need not worry about scrapes, scratches, or under-the-skin lumps that may occur when forceps have been used to assist in delivery. They too clear up in a short time.

ACTION — An infant with a collarbone fracture can be made more comfortable by pinning the sleeve of his or her undershirt across the chest, which helps immobilize the shoulder. In other birth injuries, either the delivery team will take care of problems or the problems will take care of themselves.

Bites, Animal

Biting attacks by animals that cause injury by breaking the skin.

Any cat or dog that inflicts a bite must be captured and examined by a veterinarian. The animal should be observed for ten days. If it develops signs of illness, the animal must be destroyed so the brain can be examined for signs of RABIES. Unprovoked attacks — that is, when the animal was not teased, hurt, or otherwise annoyed — cause greater concern that the animal may be rabid. Even though many pet animals are immunized, it is possible that the vaccine was ineffective or that it actually produced the disease. So the rules for confinement and observation should always be followed.

Among wild animals, skunks and bats have the highest incidence of rabies infection. Other wild meat-eating animals, including raccoons, also have a chance of becoming infected. Smaller animals — rats, rabbits, squirrels, hamsters, gerbils — seldom get the disease, but to be safe, one should check with a physician or a local emergency room whenever an animal bite occurs.

ACTION — Any breaks in the skin caused by an animal's teeth, as well as any scratches that come in contact with an animal's saliva, require prompt attention. The area should be cleansed thoroughly with soap and water and then flushed with alcohol. If the wound is large or there is significant bleeding, the child should be taken to an emergency medical facility. In some localities, any animal bite must be reported to the police.

In conjunction with the area's health department, the physician will decide what, if any, additional therapy may be needed. A decision to immunize the child with rabies vaccine depends on a number of factors, including the prevalence or absence of rabies in local animals.

The child's general immunization history should be reviewed. Children who have not had a TETANUS booster within the past five years should get one, because animal bites are notorious sites for this infectious disease. The wound must be observed carefully for redness, swelling, or drainage, indicating the presence of an infection that would require antibiotic treatment.

Bites, Human

Injuries inflicted by a person's teeth and mouth parts.

The human mouth has a remarkable variety and amount of bacterial growth that does no harm there but can cause infections if the microorganisms are driven through a break in the skin. Often this occurs in rough play or from a fist landing on someone's teeth. Depending on the site, a severe and progressive infection can develop.

Small children will sometimes bite playmates or adults out of anger. Biting the child back is not a good way to stop this behavior; neither will a slap on the face teach the child a proper way of handling anger. If you sense that the child is about to bite someone, quickly remove the child from the situation.

ACTION — Whenever skin is broken by contact with teeth, thoroughly cleanse the area with soap and water. Observe carefully for redness or swelling. If these signs develop, or if pus seeps from the wound, seek immediate medical evaluation. Antibiotic therapy is necessary and, in some cases, surgical drainage of the infection may be required. The hands are in special need of prompt treatment because tendons and other important structures may be permanently damaged from an untreated infection.

Bites, Snake

Injuries caused by the fangs and mouth parts of a snake.

Only a few snakes common to North America secrete an amount of venom sufficient to cause potentially serious problems in a child who is bitten.

There are at least two schools of thought about snakes: One recommends considering all of them possibly dangerous and to seek immediate medical attention if bitten; the other recommends learning the characteristics of poisonous snakes that inhabit the locality and being prepared to render first aid in the event that aid is not readily accessible.

Many varieties of rattlesnakes, water moccasin, and copperhead snakes are known as pit vipers because they have a pit between the eyes and nostril and on each side of the head. Their heads are rather flattened, their pupils have an elliptical shape, and they have two well-developed fangs. Two very clear puncture wounds are left where the fangs enter the skin.

Coral snakes are cobras. They have a black nose; red, black, and yellow rings around the body; and their fangs are tubular, with teeth behind the fangs. They tend to hang on to the victim, chewing into the skin. The bite of a coral snake tends to be somewhat less painful than bites by pit vipers, and there is less immediate swelling. Other than that, symptoms are similar: weakness, shortness of breath, impaired vision, rapid pulse rate, nausea, vomiting, and, in severe cases, possible shock, respiratory problems, convulsions, paralysis, and coma.

ACTION — If a child is bitten, the best treatment is immediate medical attention so that an appropriate antivenom substance can be administered. Personnel in most hospital emergency rooms no longer incise (cut) such wounds, and the effectiveness of tourniquets is in question. However, when a delay in getting modern medical treatment is unavoidable, these first-aid steps may prove valuable:

1. Immobilize the bitten area in a position lower than the heart and apply a constricting band just tight enough so that you can slip a finger under it between two and four inches above the bite, that is, between the bite and the heart.
2. Use a flame to sterilize a sharp knife, then make a short cut (no longer than half an inch) in an up-and-down direction (*not* crossways) where the venom seems to be collected, usually a bit downward from the fang marks.
3. Apply suction, if necessary, with your mouth. (The venom will not poison you if it gets in your stomach, but you should try to avoid swallowing it.) Suction should be continued for 30 minutes to an hour.
4. If swelling reaches the constricting band, add another band about two inches higher than the first one.
5. Wash the wound with soap and water and blot it dry.
6. Apply a clean bandage. Ice or cold-water applications may slow absorption of the poison — but do not pack the wound in ice.
7. Get the child to an emergency medical facility as quickly as possible. When possible, one person should drive while another continues performing the first-aid measures outlined here.

Families who like to hike, camp out, or engage in other outdoor activities that may involve encounters with poisonous snakes should buy a snakebite first-aid kit, which contains necessary materials along with instructions for use.

Bites, Spider

Injuries caused by the mouth parts of a spider.

Although most spiders in the United States are venomous and many people are bitten each year, there are only about four deaths a year.

Of the most dangerous species — black widows, brown recluse or violin spiders, jumping spiders, trap-door spiders, running spiders, tarantulas, and crab spiders — children are most bothered by the venom of the black widow and the brown recluse.

Signs and symptoms include a skin rash, itching, fever, nausea, vomiting, anxiety, sweating, weakness, and possible breathing difficulties.

ACTION — Temporary relief of pain can be achieved by placing an ice cube over the bite. No other first-aid measures are of real value, and the child should be taken to a doctor or emergency medical facility at once.

Blindness

The total absence or loss of vision.

That is the strict definition of blindness. In both the practical and legal senses, however, blindness usually includes visual defects that are so severe that certain forms of activity or eventual employment are difficult or impossible. In some cases there may be some perception of light, but the images formed on the child's retina are hazy and dim.

Causes of blindness include:

• Congenital (present-at-birth) defects of the eye, the optic nerve, or the visual center of the brain
• Wounds and other injuries
• Increased pressure within the skull
• Degeneration or detachment of the retina
• Eye or brain tumors
• Severe DIABETES MELLITUS

- MENINGITIS (an inflammation of the membranes covering the brain)
- Complications stemming from chronic inflammation of the eye

Of late there has been considerable attention paid to the disease called *retinitis pigmentosa*, which is thought to be hereditary and which eventually leads to blindness. In children who are affected, ophthalmoscopic examination by an eye doctor generally shows abnormalities by the time the child is ten years old. Poor night vision may be evident much earlier, so parents who notice that their children have unusual difficulty seeing at night should have the children's eyes examined at once.

ACTION — Some types of blindness or partial blindness can be corrected with prompt medical or surgical attention. In other cases, early treatment can arrest or slow the progress of defective eyesight that could lead to blindness. Parents should be sure that their children receive thorough eye examinations at whatever interval the pediatrician, family doctor, or health-care professional suggests.

More information on retinitis pigmentosa and blindness may be obtained by calling the following toll-free numbers: National Retinitis Pigmentosa Foundation, 800-638-2300 (301-225-9400 in Maryland); American Council of the Blind, 800-424-8666, 3 P.M. to 5:30 P.M. eastern time (202-393-3666 in Washington, D.C.); American Foundation for the Blind, 800-232-5463; Blind Children's Center, 800-222-3566.

Blisters

A raised, watery sac on the skin or the lining of the mouth.

Blisters are a reaction of the uppermost layers of the skin either to an injury from pressure or heat or to a bacterial or viral infection.

Heat injuries, including sunburn and burns and scalds, may cause extensive blistering of the skin. Pressure blisters are usually found on the hands and feet. COLD SORES (blisters on the lip) are caused by a particular virus, HERPES SIMPLEX. Occasionally an IMPETIGO may develop from a cold sore; the original spot becomes crusted and does not heal, and other sores begin to develop around the initial one.

When children run high fevers — temperatures up to 105°F (40.5°C) — blisters inside the mouth may indicate viral illnesses known as HERPETIC STOMATITIS and HERPANGIA. Despite their impressive names, neither of these diseases is serious and they usually clear up by themselves in seven to ten days. However, when the child's fever is still high and the illness is in full swing, he or she may suffer considerable pain in the throat and mouth as well as generalized aching and discomfort.

Newborn infants with a blistering type of DIAPER RASH may be infected with the *Staphylococcus* germ. And, though rare, there are several congenital (present-at-birth) skin diseases that show blistering as a predominant sign. The physician's diagnosis and subsequent treatment are based on the appearance and severity of the skin lesions.

ACTION — For heat-injury blisters: The affected areas should be cleansed with an antibacterial soap several times a day; when the injuries are extensive, they should be treated by a physician or appropriate health-care professional. Make no attempt to rupture the blister; in time the fluid will be released as the underlying skin heals. Special antibiotic creams may be necessary, and care to prevent infection is imperative.

For pressure blisters: No special care is required, except for cleansing and placing a soft dressing over the skin to prevent further injury. A nonstick pad put directly in contact with the blister allows for easy removal of any dressings.

For cold sores: The blister usually heals in eight to ten days and requires no therapy. If an IMPETIGO develops, consult the child's physician or health-care practitioner, since an oral antibiotic may be needed.

For mouth fever blisters: Parents can help by administering plenty of cool liquids and acetaminophen, and using a cotton swab to dab a soothing, nonburning preparation such as an astringent mouthwash on the blisters.

For diaper rash blisters: Prompt medical attention is necessary because of the potential need for antibiotic therapy.

Blood Poisoning

See SEPTICEMIA

Boils

A pus-filled inflammation, called a furuncle, of an infected hair follicle or sebaceous (oil-secreting) gland.

Bacteria that enter through small breaks in the skin's surface can cause many kinds of skin disorders. When they burrow through to hair roots or sebaceous glands, they may cause a walled-off area of infection that becomes red, tender, and filled with pus: a boil.

The most common sites for boils are on the face, the back of the neck, under the arms, and the lower part of the back. Cleanliness, daily changing of clothes, and the use of an antibacterial soap may reduce the likelihood of children getting boils, although some youngsters seem unusually prone to them, especially as they reach puberty, when the sebaceous glands are more active. Boils sometimes disappear spontaneously after three or four days.

ACTION — Boils should never be picked at, squeezed, or pierced at home by the parent or the child, because this may cause the bacteria, sometimes *Staphylococcus* germs, to spread to other places. Warm compresses may help bring the boil to a head and also relieve the pain.

If a boil persists or increases in size, it is best to have a physician pierce it to release the pus before a dressing is applied. In some cases, antibiotic therapy may be prescribed.

Botulism

Severe, potentially lethal form of food poisoning.

Botulism is caused by a toxin produced when the *Clostridium botulinum* bacterium grows in improperly preserved food. Symptoms include abdominal pain and vomiting, headache, general weakness, and difficulty swallowing and seeing. Death can occur when the toxin causes paralysis that strikes the nerve centers controlling breathing.

In the past few years, concern has arisen that infants may contract botulism and its serious consequences from honey that is used as a food or formula sweetener. Recent evidence suggests that commercial corn syrups may also contain the toxin in amounts harmful to babies.

ACTION — When signs of botulism occur, take the child to an emergency medical facility immediately. There, a stomach pump will be used to remove the offending food, and vomiting will be induced. The doctors will attempt to neutralize the toxin by giving the child an antitoxin medicine. They will also monitor the child's breathing and support it if necessary.

It is recommended that all home-canned foods be scrupulously checked for proper seals before serving them to anyone, and that the containers used in commercially available foods be examined for any seal problems. Further, honey or syrup sweeteners should not be fed to infants under one year of age.

Bowlegs

Bowing out of the knees, which appear too widely separated and cannot be closed when the feet are together.

Bowlegs are extremely common in infants and toddlers. The defect usually corrects itself within about one year after the child begins to walk. Sometimes there is a family history of bowlegs. Very rarely does the condition restrict or limit movement.

ACTION — The child's doctor will generally become concerned only if the condition is unusually severe or if it occurs out of its normal sequence in the growth pattern. Shoe wedges are generally not pre-scribed because they accomplish little if anything and, in fact, may make the child's feet uncomfortable.

Certain congenital (present-at-birth) diseases of bone formation as well as rickets acquired later in childhood may cause an unusual degree of bowing. On very rare occasions, a disorder known as Blount's disease causes bowlegs. The diagnosis is made by x-ray, and the defect may require bracing or even surgery for correction.

Brain Infection

See ENCEPHALITIS, MENINGITIS

Breasts, Diseases/Conditions of

Out-of-the-ordinary changes in the look, size, or feel of the breasts.

Of the various diseases/conditions of the breasts, the ones most likely to affect youngsters are:

- *Puffed-out breasts.* Newborn infants often show this condition. It is caused by the temporary hormonal influences from the mother's blood. Within a few weeks the engorgement disappears on its own.
- *Lumps under nipples.* Especially during adolescence, both girls and boys may complain of these under one or both nipples. It

occurs because tissue in that location is sensitive to normal amounts of the hormone estrogen. The area may be tender if touched or struck, but the condition is not harmful and generally disappears in a period of weeks.

- *Bleeding from the nipple.* This is almost always due to a benign (harmless) condition, but an evaluation by a physician is imperative. (Discharge from the nipple can also occur when cysts are present, but the secretions are not bloodstained.)

- *Fibroadenoma.* This is a common disease of the breast. It usually occurs during the period from puberty to 30 years of age. In young girls the tumors are firm and rubbery; they are easily moved about within the breast tissue and tend to slip away from the physician's examining fingers. They rarely grow to a large size, and they *never develop into cancer.* Neither does their occurrence increase the chances of cancer developing at a later time.

- *Mastitis.* This is the name given to an infection and inflammation of the breasts. It is most likely to occur during breast-feeding, when germs may enter through cracks babies may make when they suck on the nipples, but the disorder can occur at any age. The microorganisms that cause the infection are *Staphylococci*, the same type of germ that causes common skin infections such as BOILS.

- *Gynecomastia.* This is an abnormal enlargement of one or both male breasts. Almost half of adolescent boys experience some degree of this condition at some point after puberty. The breast may be tender at times, and there may be some enlargement of the nipples.

ACTION — For puffed out breasts: No treatment is needed, and parents can simply relax and reassure themselves that there is nothing wrong with the baby.

For lumps under nipples: Only if the area gradually enlarges need medical evaluation be sought, and then regularly scheduled checkups might be recommended.

For fibroadenoma: Treatment is the same as for any distinct lump in the breast: It may be removed surgically and examined very carefully to make absolutely sure there is no cancer involved. When the lump is removed, there is usually no disfiguration whatsoever. The scar may be barely noticeable, and recurrences are rare.

For mastitis: Antibiotics can clear up the infection within a relatively short time, especially if given early. If treatment is delayed, an abscess may form, which leads to a swelling under a reddened area of skin. If this happens, a small incision may have to be made in the breast so the fluid can be drained.

For gynecomastia: No medical treatment is needed, since the condition is harmless and disappears of its own accord within a year or two at most. However, the situation is apt to cause the adolescent enormous embarrassment, and parental reassurance in addition to a doctor's reassurance may prove helpful. Only in the rarest of instances does the overdeveloped breast tissue fail to recede; then, if the growth is excessive and causes emotional distress, surgical removal may be indicated.

Bronchiolitis

An acute inflammation of the bronchioles (the very tiny breathing tubes in the lungs) that causes a cough and wheezing.

Bronchiolitis is, in most cases, caused by a virus and is most common during the winter and early spring months. Although this disorder is seen in youngsters as old as 2 years, it usually affects babies under the age of 18 months, commonly around the age of 6 months.

The first symptoms are usually a runny nose, a low-grade fever, and other signs of an upper-respiratory infection. The cough that develops becomes progressively worse, and the child begins to wheeze. The breathing rate may increase from a normal average of 30 times per minute up to as high as 80.

Since bronchiolitis is a viral illness, not a bacterial one, antibiotics are of no value unless bacterial PNEUMONIA complicates the situation. Within a few days the wheezing lessens, and after a week to ten days the baby is well. After recovery, babies may cough for several days, but the coughing is not associated with respiratory distress.

It used to be thought that bronchiolitis would not recur in a child who had already had it. However, it now seems that babies who have had bronchiolitis do show an increased tendency to wheeze when they are stricken with other viruses that cause upper-respiratory ailments.

ACTION — A physician's evaluation is necessary because breathing distress may progress to the point at which the affected baby turns blue. Babies with bronchiolitis are often hospitalized so they can be properly oxygenated. An oxygen tent with mist allows moisture to loosen mucous secretions and makes the breathing effort easier. Hospitalization also permits professional suctioning of this mucus, as some babies tend to choke on their own secretions. In certain circumstances, an inhaled antiviral agent may be used.

Bronchitis

Inflammation of the bronchi, the large air passages that lead to the lungs. It can be chronic or acute, but acute bronchitis is more common in infants and children.

Tiredness, poor nutrition, and exposure to cold, wet, or fog seem to trigger the disease. Young children who live in damp, foggy climates are particularly susceptible. Bronchitis can be caused by infection from a virus, a bacterium, or even a fungus. In the tropics, a parasitic worm may be the culprit. It can also occur as a complication of some other illness such as PERTUSSIS (whooping cough) or MEASLES, or it may be due to an ALLERGY to irritating substances such as smoke (including cigarette smoke), dust, and some gases.

Smoking can greatly increase the risk of acute bronchitis (as well as other diseases that interfere with normal lung function), so older children experimenting with cigarette smoking should be strongly urged not to take that risk. Studies also indicate that children of parents who smoke have a higher incidence of respiratory problems.

Bronchitis strikes suddenly, and the bronchial tubes react the same way as nasal passages do to a cold: They become dry, then runny, then they gradually return to normal. The child may complain of chest discomfort that seems to be located behind the breastbone. A dry, irritating, hacking cough gradually loosens as the passages become more moist. At that time, children old enough to spit out what they cough up generally expectorate a thick, pus-tinged sputum. This is a protective mechanism and explains why most physicians are reluctant to prescribe cough syrups or antihistamines that may suppress the cough reflex.

In most instances, acute bronchitis is mild and does not last more than a few days. However, children who suffer repeated attacks should receive careful and frequent medical evaluation. Failure to take the proper measures could result in the more serious lung infection known as PNEUMONIA and could also place the child under greater risk for contracting other disorders that affect the lungs.

ACTION — Occasionally doctors may advise parents to construct "CROUP tents" over their infant's crib so that a cold-steam humidifier can moisten the air. In most cases, parents are advised merely to make sure the child gets plenty of fluids, rest, and perhaps moderate doses of acetaminophen to relieve fever — which, if present, is generally not too high. Antibiotics are not indicated unless the illness is caused or accompanied by bacterial infection.

Bronchopneumonia

See PNEUMONIA

Bulimia

An abnormal increase in the urge to eat; excessive eating.

In typical cases, the bulimic lies to others about food intake, secretly gorges on food, and then induces vomiting by sticking a finger down the throat.

More common in females than males, bulimia is thought to be associated with various underlying psychological or sociological causes, which may demand professional help. The emotional causes of bulimia are not easily resolved, but if the motivation is sufficiently strong and the victim has the understanding of the immediate family or very close friends, the outlook is promising. This condition is frequently associated with a distorted and unrealistic view of the victim's own body image and sense of personal worth.

ACTION — More information concerning bulimia, anorexia nervosa, and other eating disorders may be obtained by calling the following toll-free numbers: Bulimia-Anorexia Self-Help, 800-762-3334; Mercy Hospital Eating Disorder Unit, 800-332-2832.

See ANOREXIA NERVOSA

C

Cancer

The catchall word for various types of malignancies that have in common an abnormal, distorted, or uncontrolled growth of body cells.

In some instances, these cells are confined to a highly localized area, where the tumorous growth can be removed surgically. In many instances, metastasis (spreading) takes place; the malignant cells may be carried by the bloodstream or lymphatic system to body areas far from the original or primary site.

Of the many different malignancies, LEUKEMIA and bone cancer seem disproportionately common in children. During childhood years, the most prevalent solid tumors are the neuroblastoma, ganglioneuroma, and Wilms' tumor. The neuroblastoma and the ganglioneuroma (abnormal growths that can arise anywhere in the nervous system) can occur anywhere sympathetic nervous tissue is found, but they frequently appear as solid masses in the abdomen, most commonly occurring in the adrenal gland, which is located near the kidney. Neuroblastomas usually occur between infancy and six years.

Wilms' tumor, one of the more common malignancies of childhood, affects the kidney and usually occurs in children between six months and three years of age. Neither a neuroblastoma nor a Wilms' tumor is marked by classic symptoms that make diagnosis easy. They are generally discovered when a doctor performs a physical examination and discovers an abdominal mass. Surgery, radiation, and chemotherapy are used as treatments. Cure rates are higher for a Wilms' tumor, once considered almost invariably fatal, than for a neuroblastoma. However, when a neuroblastoma or ganglioneuroma is neatly encapsulated, surgical removal may carry a higher success rate — at least one third of children can be saved by surgery, chemotherapy, and radiation.

Cancer of the bone — in which pain is the most prominent symptom — includes giant cell sarcoma, fibrosarcoma, osteogenic sarcoma, Ewing's sarcoma, and multiple myeloma. In most instances, surgery is the primary treatment. Sometimes children may have to lose a limb, but if there has been no spread, they may survive into healthy old age.

LEUKEMIA, by far the most common cancer in children and by far the one best known to parents, is a disease in which too many underdeveloped white blood cells take over, so that the bone marrow cannot produce enough red blood cells and other elements normally present in the blood. Young children between three and five are usually the victims, although leukemia can occur at any age, through adulthood. Parents may notice a child's listlessness, paleness, proneness to infections (often with fever), and unexplained bruising (caused by heavy bleeding of small vessels).

Laboratory examination shows various abnormalities of the blood, usually including a large increase in white blood cells, but the most accurate diagnosis is made from a specialist's analysis of bone marrow. Newer forms of chemotherapy have improved the rate of remission (a time when the child is mostly free of symptoms), and now more than half of the children stricken with leukemia survive more than five years after diagnosis.

ACTION — Radiation, implantation of a radioactive substance, and chemotherapy (the administration of drugs that attack and destroy cancer cells) are common treatments for cancers, although they are frequently used in conjunction with surgery.

Supportive therapy or group talk sessions can be helpful to parents of children with any form of cancer. When the child is in remission, he or she should be allowed to engage in normal activities as long as the doctor approves.

A free brochure — *The Fight Against Childhood Cancer* — is available by writing to St. Jude Children's Research Hospital, Communications, P.O. Box 3704, Memphis, TN 38103. Enclose a self-addressed, stamped envelope.

For more information about prevention, detection, and treatment, call the following toll-free numbers: American Medical Center Cancer Information, 800-525-3777 (303-233-6501 in Colorado); American Cancer Society, 800-227-2345 from 8:30 A.M. to 4:30 P.M. eastern time; American International Hospital Cancer Program, 800-FOR

HELP; Cancer Information Service of the National Cancer Institute of the Department of Health and Human Services, 800-4-CANCER.

Candidiasis

See THRUSH, VAGINITIS, YEAST INFECTION

Canker Sores

Small painful, open ulcers (sores) that form on the lips or tissues inside the mouth that occur alone or in groups.

Canker sores are not particularly common in children, although when they do appear they tend to recur (as happens with adults). The cause may be connected to dietary deficiencies, particularly vitamin B_{12} and folic acid; allergies; infectious microorganisms; or emotional stress, although most often no cause can be determined. It is not a serious condition, although it may temporarily interfere with a child's eating habits.

ACTION — Canker sores ordinarily heal by themselves within one or two weeks. If the child is particularly bothered by the pain and discomfort, a physician may prescribe a painkiller that can be applied directly to the sore.

Carbuncle

A bacterial skin infection caused by Staphylococcus *bacteria.*

Carbuncles look like a collection of BOILS, except that the infection extends over a wide area, affects deeper layers of the skin, and takes longer to heal than do boils.

ACTION — Because of the seriousness of the infections, carbuncles should receive prompt medical attention. The doctor may suggest the use of warm compresses, which help stimulate an adequate blood supply and bring an infected lesion to a head. Doctors usually treat carbuncles by lancing and draining the lesion and prescribing an antibiotic. Parents should discard all soiled compresses or dressings to prevent possible infection of other family members.

Celiac Disease

See MALABSORPTION SYNDROME

Cerebral Palsy

A condition primarily affecting motor development, muscular control, and coordination, caused by damage to the brain.

Damage to the brain that causes cerebral palsy may occur during or just before birth, but may also take place in early infancy; approximately 2 out of every 1,000 newborns are afflicted. It is often not easy to tell from child to child the exact cause of their cerebral palsy; some of the possible causes have to do with diseases or conditions involving the mother, and nearly all have to do with lack of oxygen to the child's brain due to the mother's alcoholism or drug addiction, RUBELLA, maternal infections, and genetic factors, among others. That a baby is born prematurely may also have much to do with acquiring cerebral palsy. When cerebral palsy develops later in early childhood, strokes, head injuries, and damage from infections are among the chief culprits.

Symptoms of cerebral palsy — which is usually recognized and diagnosed before the age of five — include defects in speech and hearing, spastic paralysis, mental retardation, and seizures. Movement is awkward at best, impossible at worst, and the arms are more affected than the legs.

ACTION — Children with cerebral palsy can benefit from physical therapy as well as speech and occupational therapies. Braces to help them with muscle control may also be ordered, and orthopedic surgery is also a possible recommendation. Muscle stiffness and spasticity can be alleviated by specific prescribed medications. It is best to start therapies early on, but even if delayed, they can still produce excellent results.

For more information about this condition and support groups, call the toll-free number of the United Cerebral Palsy Association, 800-USA-1UCP.

Chicken Pox

A highly contagious and infectious disease caused by a herpes virus called varicella.

Infants up to about the age of six months are thought to possess natural immunity to chicken pox, although they may contract the disease in unusual circumstances; a breast-fed baby, whose mother has had chicken pox and whose milk contains the antibody, may be protected even further. Peak incidence occurs between the ages of five and nine, although older children and even adults can be infected — and from the age of ten onward the victim feels more ill.

The incubation period is about 14 days, although it may range from 11 to 20 days, after which time spots begin to appear all over the body, sometimes even inside the cheeks, on the roof of the mouth, or on the scalp, although they tend to be concentrated mostly on the chest, back, and upper thighs. The spots appear in crops, beginning as small pink marks. Within just a few hours the spots turn into tiny blisters and look like drops of water resting on the skin. They vary in size from that of a pinhead to a split pea. The blisters then cloud over and form a crust. Sometime after 10 to 20 days the crusty scabs fall away and leave pink marks. These marks eventually disappear entirely; parents can be reassured that scarring is rare.

The main discomfort of chicken pox comes from the itching. It is important to keep the child from scratching or picking at the scabs — not, contrary to common belief, because it spreads the disease itself, which is viral and blood-borne, but because opening the skin may provide a route for infection by bacteria or do enough damage to scar the skin.

Younger children ill with chicken pox usually have just a slight fever at first; they rarely feel ill enough to remain in bed more than four or five days and need not remain in bed at all unless they wish to. Children should be kept isolated for about one week after the rash appears; they are infectious as long as new crops of lesions are developing. The contagious period ranges from one or two days before the rash appears to about seven days after its onset.

ACTION — When the rash of chicken pox first appears, parents should tell the doctor so he or she can confirm the diagnosis and recommend appropriate itch-relieving medications, some of which can be taken orally (for example, pediatric forms of Benadryl and Atarax) and others which are applied directly to the skin. Cool baths also help relieve itching; there are several commercial bath lotions that may be soothing, as well as home remedies such as adding cornstarch to the bath. Chicken pox is essentially a home-treatable disease unless the child has LEUKEMIA or some other serious disorder that affects the body's immune system, in which case special medical attention is required to prevent serious side effects of this usually mild childhood illness.

See and compare MEASLES

Chinese Restaurant Syndrome

Allergic reaction to ingestion of monosodium glutamate (MSG).

Monosodium glutamate (MSG), a flavor enhancer, is used to a large extent in Chinese food. Upon eating food containing this additive, sensitive children (and adults too) experience frightening but essentially harmless symptoms, including a throbbing head (feeling as if it is expanding and contracting, which is what the MSG is doing to the arteries), dizziness, an unusual pinpricking feeling, and tightness around the jaw, throat, and upper back.

ACTION — Nearly all of the time, simply comforting the child and letting the symptoms run their relatively brief course are all that is required. If the child is extremely frightened or seems to be in physical distress, immediate medical attention is warranted. Prevention is the best cure; avoid adding MSG to foods cooked at home, and always ask about such additives when eating out. Many Chinese and other restaurants offer dishes made without MSG.

Cholesterol, High Levels of

See HYPERCHOLESTEREMIA

Chorea

A nervous disorder characterized by involuntary muscular twitching and irregular jerky movements.

Sydenham's chorea, also known as St. Vitus' dance, can occur as a complication of streptococcal infections and is sometimes associated with RHEUMATIC FEVER. The condition, more common in girls than in boys, usually subsides within about three months — six to eight months at the most.

A diagnosis of Huntington's chorea is far more serious. It is a hereditary disease that eventually leads to mental deterioration, although symptoms usually do not occur until victims are in their mid-thirties. However, the genetic possibility of transmission is so high that authorities advise members of any family with a known history of the disease not to have children.

ACTION — A sedative or tranquilizer can be helpful in some cases of Sydenham's chorea. Parents need not be unduly concerned, and children should be given plenty of reassurance that the condition is temporary and there will be no lasting physical effects and no damage to the mind.

However, since people without medical training are not in a position to assess children's twitching, clumsiness, or impaired muscular coordination (in some instances, children subconsciously or unconsciously display unusual arm, leg, or facial movements because of psychological stress), parents should take any child showing these symptoms to a doctor.

More information about Huntington's chorea may be obtained by calling the toll-free number of the Huntington's Disease Society of America at 800-345-4372 (212-242-1968 in New York City).

Cleft Lip/Cleft Palate

A congenital (present-at-birth) deformity manifesting itself as a split of the lip and/or roof of the mouth.

In this birth defect affecting fewer than 3 in 1,000 children, the face may not form properly. This may involve just the outer, visible portion of the lip area (often called *harelip*) or may involve the entire upper jaw, creating a fissure from front to back. Frequently cleft lip or palate may accompany other birth defects in a child. There may be a genetic component to the condition.

Breast-feeding or use of a nippled bottle is difficult if not impossible for infants with cleft palates. Even when liquid nourishment is fed to the child by using a cup or some other device, the child still experiences difficulty because the liquid can enter the nose through the cleft, causing choking and other discomfort. Later, the distorted palate will cause speech defects.

ACTION — Cleft lip and palate can be corrected by reconstructive surgery: The lip should be taken care of when the child is about 2 or 3 months old, while the palate operation should be performed before the child reaches the age of 18 months. Successful surgery leaves very little scarring. Speech therapy may still be required to help the child develop a normal speaking voice with few impediments, while dental and hearing problems may need to be looked at and treated.

For more information, the American Cleft Palate Educational Foundation offers a toll-free number: 800-24-CLEFT.

Clubfoot

A congenital (present-at-birth) abnormality in which the heel is high and the foot and toes point downward and inward.

Clubfoot is not too common a disorder, occurring in somewhat less than 1 out of every 1,000 births, and it is sometimes accompanied by other malformations (for example, lack of proper closure in the bony segments around the spinal cord). It is somewhat more common in males than females and may occur more frequently in the case of multiple births.

ACTION — Treatment usually consists of applying a series of casts that allow gradual movement of the foot back into its normal position. Later, corrective shoes are worn until the growth period ends. In less severe cases, splinting may correct the abnormality, and in more severe cases surgical correction may be required.

Cold

See COMMON COLD

Cold Sore

A localized infection caused by the HERPES SIMPLEX *virus, Type I.*

A cold sore sometimes accompanies the COMMON COLD, is often recurrent, and characteristically develops into a small group of fever blisters, especially around the lips and at the corners of the mouth.

ACTION — The discomfort of cold sores can sometimes be relieved by the application of skin balms, lotions, or glycerin-type preparations. Parents of children who suffer persistent bouts of cold sores may wish to have a doctor check the lesion to make sure it is not a bacterial infection such as IMPETIGO.

See also BLISTERS, HERPES SIMPLEX

Colitis

An inflammation of the colon (the large intestine). It may be related to a wide range of underlying conditions, such as AMEBIC DYSENTERY *and* BACILLARY DYSENTERY.

Colitis is not particularly prevalent in childhood; its highest incidence occurs between the ages of 15 and 40. In addition to inflammation, ulcerative colitis involves ulceration of the mucous membrane that lines the large intestine. The condition is marked by acute AB-DOMINAL PAIN and the frequent passage of foul-smelling, watery stools that contain blood, mucus, and pus. Sometimes the disease begins with a sudden and violent attack of bloody diarrhea and high fever of 103° to 104°F.

ACTION — Immediate medical attention is essential at the first suggestion of ulcerative colitis, because severe, rapidly progressive first attacks can be life threatening.

Collapsed Lung

See PNEUMOTHORAX

Color Blindness

A deficiency of vision in which one cannot differentiate between certain colors, usually red and green.

In most cases, the color-sensitive receptors (called cones) of the retina in the eye that distinguish colors malfunction or are damaged, leading to a child's inability to see those colors clearly or to tell them apart. It is mainly a hereditary condition affecting boys (caused by a gene passed down by the mother), although diseases and injuries can lead to the problem. *Monochromatism*, in which no colors at all can be distinguished, is extremely rare.

ACTION — There is no known cure for color blindness, which is a lifelong condition. It is seldom a problem, although it may limit career choices — because some occupations require the worker to distinguish a red electrical wire, say, from a green one — make the appreciation of art difficult and frustrating, and create occasionally embarrassing clothing color combinations. Aside from these and a few other minor life-style glitches, color blindness is easily accommodated by children.

Common Cold

A highly contagious acute viral infection of the upper-respiratory tract.

Viruses, the smallest known particles capable of causing disease, are responsible for the common cold. A cold can be caused by any one of more than a hundred different viruses, which is why many children, and adults, seem to have colds that last all winter: They suffer from one infection after another.

Colds are spread by the viruses simply floating through the air from one child's nose and mouth to another child's nose and mouth. Crowding indoors, such as in day-care and school settings, makes infection almost impossible to avoid. The frequency of colds in young children probably builds future immunity. This explains why young children can normally be expected to get up to eight colds each year, while adolescents average only two to four a year.

Symptoms usually include chills, sore throat, runny nose, stuffy nose (nasal congestion), slight headache, and, sometimes, a cough and fever. Colds usually last from three to seven days.

ACTION — Since viruses do not respond to antibiotics or to other drugs that fight bacteria, treatment remains geared to relieving discomfort and being prudent about exposing others to the cold virus. Keep the child home at least three days — the contagious period. A humidifier may relieve the congestion and coughing, which are often particularly bad at night. Drinking lots of liquids helps thin mucous secretions, and older children should cut back on milk, which tends to thicken these secretions. When giving children nonprescription drugs such as aspirinlike compounds, nose drops or sprays, or preparations that soothe throats and lessen coughing, always follow label directions carefully.

Normally, children do not need a doctor's evaluation unless there are complications such as a persisting temperature of over 102°F; a cough that produces thick, discolored material; swollen glands; pain in the teeth or a severe headache; discoloring of the nails, skin, or lips;

and any marked change in the child's normal behavior pattern. On occasion a bad cold may lead to SINUSITIS (inflammation of the sinuses), EAR INFECTIONS, or BRONCHITIS.

Concussion

A violent jarring of the brain, a cerebral concussion is caused by a blow to the head or a head injury such as might occur when a child falls.

The trauma may seem insignificant, but the damage may be severe. Dizziness, headaches, and vomiting may be dominant symptoms of concussion. Return of full consciousness is gradual, although it usually takes only a few minutes.

Parents should remain alert to the following signs that may follow a concussion. If they occur, the doctor should be notified immediately, or the child should be taken for emergency medical assessment.

1. Nonuse of an arm or leg
2. Convulsions
3. Inequality in the size of the pupils of the eyes
4. Repeated vomiting
5. Unusual behavior
6. Difficulty in arousing the child

Parents used to be advised to keep the child awake, but it is now considered sufficient to awaken concussion victims every two hours to check for these abnormalities.

ACTION — Whenever parents have the slightest cause to suspect that a child has sustained a concussion, or if the child has been unconscious even briefly, they should notify a doctor immediately. Prompt medical evaluation and perhaps x-rays will be needed to ensure that there is no skull fracture or any rupture of blood vessels within the brain.

Hospitalization may or may not be necessary; it depends on the results of the physician's neurological examination. If the child soon regains normal alertness, doctors have discovered no signs or symptoms of potentially serious brain damage, and the parents can be counted on to be watchful, the youngster may be allowed to go home.

Conjunctivitis

An inflammation of the conjunctiva (the membrane that lines the eyelid and covers the white of the eye). Commonly called "pinkeye."

In rare instances, conjunctivitis is caused by a newborn infant's reaction to silver nitrate, a chemical instilled at the time of delivery. In even rarer instances, a newborn infant's conjunctivitis may occur because silver nitrate is *not* instilled and the mother has gonorrhea. Less infrequently, the condition may be a reaction to specks of dirt or other foreign objects. By far the most common cause of pinkeye is bacterial or viral infections that are highly contagious and seem to appear in epidemics.

The first signs of conjunctivitis are usually a burning or smarting sensation of the eyelids, along with intense itching. The white of the eye becomes pink or bright red, and the eye waters excessively. This watery discharge may change to a sticky secretion containing pus, which causes the eyelashes and eyelids to stick together, especially when the child sleeps. The lids often become swollen, and in severe cases both eyes are involved.

ACTION — Mild forms of pinkeye usually clear up within a few days, especially if the outsides of the eyes are gently and regularly bathed in warm water. It is wisest, however, to check with the child's physician so that eyedrops can be prescribed as required by the condition.

If the parent seeks medical advice and the doctor prescribes an antibiotic ointment, be careful to apply the medication correctly. An ointment is spread in a thin line along the lower eyelid, which is retracted (held down). Use of eyedrops is often restricted to older children because of difficulties that even the most dedicated parent may experience when trying to instill drops into a squirming youngster's eye.

When pinkeye is severe or tends to recur frequently, the child should be examined and treated by a doctor or qualified health-care professional.

Convulsive Disorders

See SEIZURE DISORDERS

Cradle Cap

Popular term for a distinctive seborrheic dermatitis

Cradle cap is a skin inflammation that produces thick, yellowish, scaly crusts and occurs in infants between birth and six months, usually clearing up by the time they are a year old.

Cradle cap is generally most prominent on the scalp, although sometimes other areas, such as the eyebrows, ears, armpits, and diaper areas, are affected.

ACTION — Mild cases can often be controlled simply by vigorously washing the scalp with soap and water, then gently scraping away all the scales with a soft brush or fine-toothed comb. Parents need not be afraid of damaging the fontanel (soft spot); the area is pliable but dense, and the pressure of a good shampooing will do no damage.

In more persistent cases, the child's physician may prescribe a corticosteroid preparation or a sulfur ointment in addition to a special medicated shampoo. Once the scalp condition clears, any associated body rashes also clear up.

Do not apply baby oil, as it only aggravates the condition, which is caused by a buildup of natural body oils.

Cretinism

See THYROID DISORDERS

Cross-Eye

See STRABISMUS

Croup

A general term that describes a distinctly resonant, barking cough usually accompanied by difficulty in breathing and hoarseness.

Croup occurs when there is a spasm or obstruction of the larynx (the voice box). Most often it is caused by an acute viral infection of the upper and lower parts of the respiratory tract, but it may also occur as

a complication of LARYNGITIS, PERTUSSIS (whooping cough), or DIPH-
THERIA, or because of an ALLERGY or the presence of a foreign body in
the larynx.

Children from about three months to seven years are most susceptible to croup, and the malady usually strikes during winter months.

In most instances, croup presents no real threat, even though an
attack may be as alarming to the parents as it is to the child. Usually
these children have colds. They wake up at night because a trickle of
mucus or other discharge has irritated and blocked the larynx, causing it to go into a brief spasm. This temporarily interferes with normal
breathing and the child has a violent attack of coughing. The hoarse
cough and the sudden wakening with a breathing difficulty are frightening. The fright may cause the spasms to worsen. If parents panic,
the situation tends to worsen. Gentle reassurance and perhaps a cup
of cocoa or some other drink that is special to the child can ease the
child's anxiety. A good way to assess severity is to note whether the
child is croupy only when coughing or whether noisy breathing continues when the child is resting. If the noise continues, the child
should be seen by a doctor or qualified health-care professional.

Croup caused by viral infection may last for three days or so. An
extremely severe and dangerous form of croup is called epiglottitis.
Children with this disease very rapidly develop difficulty breathing,
perhaps even turning blue in a matter of a few hours. High fever is
present, and the child looks very ill. Swallowing is so painful that
children with epiglottitis cannot swallow their own saliva, so they
drool. They also want to sit upright and lean forward, a natural defense against complete closure of the airway.

ACTION — Children should be kept comfortable and given plenty to
drink. Home treatment can be provided by using cold-steam humidi-
fiers or steam from a hot tub or shower. The parent should stay with
the child when the bathroom door is shut to allow steam to accumulate. Exposure to the steam should be limited to ten minutes. If the
croup is not relieved by steam inhalation, medical attention should be
sought.

Particularly in very small children, marked respiratory distress or
other problems may require hospitalization so that these children can
be under constant observation and be given oxygen. In severe cases,
the air passages may become obstructed with a membrane, swelling,
or thick mucus so that a tracheotomy (cutting a temporary air passage
into the throat) may be necessary.

A child with severe croup needs immediate emergency medical attention.

Cystic Fibrosis

An inherited, fatal disease involving a general dysfunction of the exocrine glands, which occurs in about 1 in every 2,000 live births, primarily among Caucasian children.

This dysfunction leads to thick secretions that clog mucous glands lining the respiratory tract. These thick, mucuslike secretions also obstruct the pancreas duct system so that enzymes necessary for proper digestion and absorption fail to operate. Sweat glands also malfunction.

Researchers have recently discovered and isolated the protein-related gene that causes cystic fibrosis, which affects about 30,000 people in the United States (1,000 to 1,200 new cases each year). Although a parent having the defective cystic fibrosis gene is a "carrier" of the disease, both parents must have the gene in order to pass it on to a child, who has a 25 percent chance of getting it.

The disease usually begins in infancy. The child tends to have chronic respiratory infections and a lack of tolerance for heat; excessive sweating is common. Occasionally there is an obstruction of the small intestine during the first few days of life because of thick greenish meconium (a substance created in the baby's intestinal tract while the infant is in the uterus).

By the age of about one year, about 80 percent of children affected show disturbances in breathing or digestion. Coughing is the most troublesome symptom during the early stages of the disease, and at first it may be mistaken for whooping cough. Episodes of vomiting also occur. Older infants and children have steatorrhea (excessive amounts of fat in bowel movements). Older children may sweat profusely, which can lead to a severe loss of essential body fluids and salts. Unless this situation is corrected by appropriate therapy, the child may suffer dehydration and circulatory failure.

ACTION — There is no known cure for cystic fibrosis. However, aggressive medical treatment can offer the child some relief through drainage of pus-filled mucous secretions from the respiratory tract, the use of pancreatic enzymes to help the gastrointestinal tract digest nutrients, antibiotics to ward off lung infections, and supervised vitamin therapy.

Professional help can be extended to the parents, who may want genetic counseling about having other children as well as assistance in dealing with the fact that their child has a potentially fatal disease.

Additional information about these matters and about the disease itself can be obtained from the Cystic Fibrosis Foundation, which can be reached at the following toll-free number between the hours of 8:30 A.M. and 5 P.M. eastern time: 800-FIGHT-CF (301-951-4422 in Maryland).

Cystitis

Inflammation of the urinary bladder, usually caused by a bacterial infection.

Although it is not a common disease of childhood, cystitis tends to occur somewhat more often in girls, because the female urethra (the passageway leading from the bladder to the outside opening) is much shorter than in males and provides easier access for infectious organisms.

The disease may be acute or chronic. In the acute form, the young person typically complains of painful urination and the frequent urge to pass urine even though the bladder may be empty. Freshly passed urine is clouded in appearance, because of the presence of pus, and often has a strong fishy odor. A steady dull ache may be experienced in the lower part of the abdomen, which is quite sensitive to the slightest pressure. Sometimes the urethra is also inflamed (urethritis), and in severe forms of cystitis the patient may have a high fever (102°F) and sweat profusely.

The diagnosis can be confirmed by laboratory tests involving urine bacterial counts. Other measures, such as x-rays to make sure the infection is not related to a structural defect or obstruction of the urinary system, may be necessary. The doctor must also make sure that the infection is, in fact, restricted to the bladder and has not spread upward to the kidneys. Sometimes a urologist (a doctor specializing in diseases of the urinary system) will use a special instrument called a cystoscope to inspect the inside of the urethra and bladder.

ACTION — Successful treatment involves the early administration of an appropriate antibiotic, drinking lots of water and other fluids, and restricting intake of spicy foods or other substances that might irritate the bladder after they are filtered to become part of the urine. Follow-up bacterial counts are usually taken to confirm recovery.

D

Deafness

Complete or partial loss of the ability to hear in one or both ears.

Deafness may be caused by any one of several factors, including infection, and the hearing loss may be only temporary (as rarely occurs with too much ear wax) or permanent (as in congenital deafness).

There are two basic classifications: *conductive deafness* and *nerve deafness*. Conductive deafness occurs when there is any interference with sound vibrations during their passage to the inner ear. In the outer passage, this interference could be caused by an infection that discharges obstructive fluid; swelling and closure of the passage, or, less commonly, excessive ear wax. In the so-called middle ear, inflammation or an obstructing growth of tissue or bone could cause deafness. Enlargement of a child's adenoids or similar lymph tissue at the back of the throat can block the opening of the eustachian tube (a short canal that connects this region with the middle ear); this blockage disturbs air pressure and reduces hearing. Rupture, inflammation, or scarring can affect the eardrum itself.

Nerve deafness, sometimes called perceptive deafness, is the most common cause of total and permanent deafness. It is sometimes a complication of some disease or injury that affects the cochlea (where sound vibrations are transformed into nerve impulses) or the auditory nerve (which transmits impulses to the brain).

Congenital deafness (deafness present from birth) is a rather rare condition for which the cause often remains unknown. Sometimes it may be connected to the mother having had RUBELLA (German measles) during early pregnancy.

Observant parents note very early on if their child is not responding to speech, the clapping of hands, sudden noises, and normal household noises. A newborn infant should show the "startle response" to a sudden loud noise, and infants as young as three months can be tested by sophisticated audiometric (hearing-measuring) techniques.

Parents who suspect some hearing deficiency in a child who is six to eight months old can try clapping their hands behind the child's head where he or she *cannot see the action*. This is important because a youngster sometimes learns to interpret the movements and gestures of the parents to compensate for unheard speech. Thus deafness can sometimes go undetected for two or three years — although if by that time the child is not speaking at least a few words that are correct and distinctly pronounced, parents should be suspicious, since deaf children cannot learn to imitate speech they do not hear.

ACTION — Early medical evaluation is essential, for if children are not properly diagnosed and, when possible, treated, they may suffer irreparable psychological damage from being categorized by their peers, schoolmates, teachers, and others as being slow, dumb, or stupid. Sometimes the removal of hardened and impacted ear wax is all that is needed. Various types of hearing aids (body aids, eyeglass aids, aids in the ear itself) can sometimes be used as early as the age of nine months. Many kinds of conductive deafness can be corrected surgically. If the child suffers permanent nerve deafness, he or she will need special training to learn to capitalize on other senses that are intact.

More information may be obtained by calling the following toll-free numbers: Better Hearing Institute, 800-424-8576 or 800-EAR-WELL, Monday through Friday, 9 A.M. to 5 P.M. eastern time (703-642-0580 in Virginia); Deafness Research Foundation, 800-535-3323; Hearing Aid Help Line, 800-521-5247, 9 A.M. to 5 P.M. eastern time; Hearing Screening Test (on-line hearing test), 800-222-EARS, Monday through Friday, 9 A.M. to 6 P.M. eastern time (800-345-3277 in Pennsylvania); National Association for Hearing and Speech, 800-638-8255 (301-897-8682 in Maryland); TRIPOD Grapevine, 800-352-8888, 8 A.M. to 6 P.M. Pacific time.

Depression

An emotional state characterized by an intense feeling of sadness, believed to occur because of feelings of loss or lack of love, although chemical imbalances may cause what is termed biologic depression.

Depression was formerly thought to be basically an adult disease, but experts in the field now realize that it is not all that rare in children, especially school-age children and adolescents. Even infants can feel sad, which is usually signaled by poor weight gain and a general lack of response to the environment.

Parents should be particularly aware of BEHAVIOR CHANGES in the child. They may note symptoms such as sleep disturbances, tearfulness, poor appetite, and low energy levels. There may be a withdrawal from social activities or a faltering academic performance in school. Sometimes other behaviors, such as anxiety reactions, AGGRESSIVE BEHAVIOR, TEMPER TANTRUM, HYPERACTIVE BEHAVIOR, RESTLESS BEHAVIOR, complaints of HEADACHE or ABDOMINAL PAIN, or just plain misbehavior or constant clowning around, may mask the depressive state. Eventually, the feelings may become so intense that they interfere with the child's day-to-day activities; personal hygiene or performance of simple everyday tasks may suffer. When such changes occur, it is best not to punish the child; neither is it appropriate to try to encourage an unrealistic sense of optimism.

ACTION — If parents cannot understand what is going on and cannot help their depressed children work through the depression, and a physician can find no biological basis for the depression, it is advisable to seek a professional psychological evaluation. This is, of course, mandatory should the young person be preoccupied with thoughts about death or SUICIDE. Parents should be particularly sensitive to a depressed adolescent suddenly becoming overly joyful; sometimes this signals a resolve to commit suicide.

Diabetes Mellitus

A disorder associated with a faulty metabolism of carbohydrates.

In diabetes mellitus, certain cells in the pancreas, called the islet of Langerhans, fail to secrete enough insulin, a hormone circulated in the bloodstream that regulates sugar metabolism. Why diabetes mellitus occurs remains unknown, but authorities have considerable evidence to indicate that the disease is hereditary.

Approximately 40 in every 10,000 children have diabetes mellitus. Unlike adults, who often experience a gradual onset after many years of a prediabetic condition, children often manifest the disease rather suddenly and often more severely. Early signs include weight loss; frequent passing of urine; an almost unquenchable thirst and hunger; itchy, dry skin; and weakness and fatigue. Later, additional symptoms often include difficulty in breathing; extreme fatigue; and gastrointestinal problems such as loss of appetite, abdominal pain, and vomiting.

If the child remains untreated, the gradual accumulation of sugar in the blood may result in what is known as a diabetic coma. In such a state, the child loses consciousness and may not survive without prompt medical or first-aid treatment. Warning signs may include nausea (often followed by vomiting), drowsiness, dry mouth, and deepened breathing before the child passes out. The situation can be confused with coma or the state of shock brought on by HYPOGLYCEMIA (low blood sugar), which sometimes occurs when an overdose of insulin depletes the blood-sugar level too suddenly.

Early medical assessment is needed so that appropriate treatment can be started with the diabetic child. A simple urine test may show glycosuria (too much sugar, in the form of glucose, in the urine). Blood samples may also be taken to see how well the patient tolerates glucose. Sometimes chemicals called ketones are present, and they often give a child's breath and urine an almost sickeningly sweet smell.

In the past, diabetic children on insulin were advised to restrict sugar, starch, and other carbohydrates. However, most doctors now contend that diabetic children should be allowed to eat what the family eats, within reason. This may be particularly so with adolescents, who are apt to regard strict dietary rules as yet another interference with their growing independence — and one they are especially apt to ignore.

Heavy exercise tends to decrease the blood-sugar level, so children hard at play may require less insulin than usual. But all diabetic patients should carry with them an emergency supply of sugar to take when they sense that their blood-sugar level is falling. The symptoms are restlessness, confusion, faintness, cold perspiration, hunger, and muscular unsteadiness. It is a good idea for the child's friends to know the signs and symptoms of lowered blood-sugar levels so that they, as well as the family, can help monitor the diabetic's condition.

Research into the control and cure of diabetes mellitus is exciting and ground breaking, and many doctors feel that whether through implants or transplants, diabetes may be tamed in the not-so-distant future.

ACTION — In most cases, children with diabetes are treated with daily injections of insulin. Older children are instructed how to administer these shots and how to do finger-stick blood tests so that they can adjust the daily dose if the need arises. Younger children's parents are given the same instructions.

Diabetic children should be checked frequently by their doctors, as a number of complications can occur. Checkups should include regular routine eye examinations to prevent a condition known as *diabetic retinopathy*, in which ruptured blood vessels can cause a swelling of the retina and gradual loss of vision.

With modern forms of treatment, the lives of diabetics are far less restricted and confining than they once were. Careful home monitoring of sugar levels prevents later development of complications affecting organs such as the kidneys or eyes. To the extent that the doctor allows, parents should try not to be overprotective. Otherwise children with diabetes may develop emotional blocks about their own capacity to compete, have fun, and live lives that are essentially normal except for daily medication, keeping tabs on their condition, and seeing doctors more frequently than most people do.

For more information about the disease, its treatment, and referrals to physicians, clinics, and support groups, call the following toll-free numbers: American Diabetes Association, 800-232-3472 between 8:30 A.M. and 5 P.M. eastern time; Juvenile Diabetes Foundation Hot Line, 800-223-1138 (212-889-7575 in New York City).

Diaper Rash

A term describing a group of red, inflamed, often raw rashes that at one time or another affect the bottom, abdomen, and inner thighs of just about all infants and small children who wear diapers.

The most common reason for these rashes is the simple mechanical action of wetness — from perspiration, urine, or stool — combined with the friction diapers make as the baby moves. Many culprits have been named: bacteria and funguses; the ammonia content of urine; chemicals found in soaps, detergents, and disposable diapers. It is impossible to control all the factors that may cause diaper rash.

Once the skin is broken, a bacterial or fungal infection can set in. Newborns are especially susceptible to staphylococcal infections that show as small pus-filled eruptions with bright red bases. A bright red rash with small pinpoint-size red spots around the margin may indicate candidiasis or THRUSH (a monilial infection), which requires prescription medication. If signs such as these occur or the diaper rash fails to clear within three or four days, the child should be checked by a doctor or qualified health-care professional for an accurate diagnosis and an effective treatment.

ACTION — Most diaper rashes clear up spontaneously and do not require any heroic measures on the part of the parents or doctor. Sometimes the baby's doctor prescribes a special ointment, especially if a fungal rash is caused by *Monilia.*

Gentle cleansing with cotton and mild soap, followed by thorough drying, is important. When the diaper can be left off completely, there is less moisture to contend with. At night the baby can sleep on a pile of diapers; this should leave much of the area free of wetness. When diapers are used, they should be loose-fitting cotton and worn without plastic overpants until the rash has cleared.

Once the rash is better, disposable diapers or plastic pants can be used again. Heavy talcum powders should be avoided because they increase friction. Dusting powders, including the medicated ones, may be helpful, and a topical cortisone cream greatly reduces inflammation. As with all medications, read and follow label instructions carefully.

If there are open, weeping spots, parents can apply compresses of salt solution: one level teaspoonful of salt to a pint of water that has been boiled, then cooled to room temperature. The compresses can be applied four times a day for ten minutes each time.

Diphtheria

A potentially serious contagious disease caused by Corynebacterium diphtheriae, *a germ that infects the back of the nose and throat, resulting in a grayish-white membrane that clogs the throat and interferes with breathing.*

Formerly a great scourge among infants and young children, diphtheria has been almost eradicated by the introduction of a protective vaccine called DPT. It is unlikely that today's parents will ever encounter the disease. However, in a few instances, immunization may have been inadequate. The disease is highly contagious and may result in severe complications if the antitoxin is not administered promptly.

ACTION — If the child shows a particularly sore throat, difficulty in swallowing, extreme weakness (which can result if the diphtheria toxin is released into the body), and breathing difficulties, be sure to check with the child's doctor.

Down's Syndrome

A genetically determined congenital condition that manifests itself with facial malformations and mental retardation.

Every cell in the body carries chromosomes, microscopic rod-shaped substances that carry hereditary features. Normally every cell in the human male and female carries 23 pairs of chromosomes for a total of 46. In Down's syndrome, there is an extra chromosome 21, called trisomy 21, so a Down's syndrome child has 47 chromosomes in each cell. Typically such children are born to women over the age of 35 and especially over the age of 40. Yet the disorder can occur in children of younger women, and in approximately one third of cases studied the extra chromosome 21 comes from the father.

The child with Down's syndrome is born with a small and slightly flattened head; distinctive facial characteristics that include slanted eyes (hence the old term "mongolism"), a flat-bridged nose, and a large tongue that tends to protrude; a lack of muscle coordination; short and stubby hands and feet; and varying degrees of mental retardation and slowed physical growth.

In addition to these abnormalities, many Down's syndrome children have heart defects, and they seem especially prone to develop LEUKEMIA. Therefore, life expectancy is not very great, although some sufferers do survive into adulthood.

Infants with Down's syndrome rarely cry; they seem quiet and peaceful, show poor muscle tone and little activity, and tend to display little interest in objects and activities that usually fascinate babies.

ACTION — Studies show that children with Down's syndrome who are raised at home usually develop more skills than those who are institutionalized at a very young age, but family circumstances may play a large role in determining if, and when, parents elect to place their child in an appropriate caretaking/educational setting.

Modern advances in prebirth detection may be of help to concerned parents-to-be. *Amniocentesis*, a process by which a sample of intra-uterine fluid is extracted from a pregnant woman, tells doctors whether the fetus has Down's syndrome. This allows parents to consider the possible early termination of a pregnancy and also to decide whether they should confer with a genetic counselor, who may help them arrive at a decision about not having, or having, other children.

More information about Down's syndrome can be obtained by calling the following toll-free numbers: National Down's Syndrome Congress, 800-232-6372; National Down's Syndrome Society, 800-221-4602 (212-460-9330 in New York City).

Dysentery

See AMEBIC DYSENTERY, BACILLARY DYSENTERY

E

Ear Infections

Infections affecting the outer, middle, or inner portion of the ear.

Most children seem unusually prone to ear infections. Because the three separate portions of the human ear may show different kinds of infections and their related symptoms, parents need to know a little bit about these anatomical areas. The outermost portion of the outer ear canal is visible. It is a tubelike structure that leads inward to a thin membrane called the eardrum. Sound waves pass from here into the middle ear, where small bones work to further transmit sound and where the eustachian tube helps equalize air pressure. In the inner ear lie structures that convert sound waves into nerve impulses (to be transferred to the brain for processing) and help maintain a person's sense of equilibrium or balance.

Otitis externa (outer ear infection) may occur when a child gets water in his or her ear that carries bacteria or fungi and does not dry completely. The lining of the canal swells and drains and becomes quite painful. Fever or nasal congestion is rarely present, but the child complains vigorously if the ear is pressed or the earlobe is tugged.

Otitis media (middle ear infection) is more frequent; few children and adolescents seem to escape at least one bout. Blockage of the eustachian tube is a common cause. Usually a middle ear infection is preceded by signs of a common cold with nasal congestion and cough. Approximately 60 percent of the time a fever is present, with temperatures over 101°F (38.3°C).

Otitis interna or *labyrinthitis* (inner ear infection) is not common during childhood. On occasion it may occur when infection spreads inward from the middle ear or downward from the meninges (the three membranes that cover the brain). Sometimes an inner ear infection may be associated with INFLUENZA. Common signs are dizziness (vertigo), TINNITUS (ringing in the ear), and partial or total loss of hearing in the affected ear. Symptoms are frequently worse when the child makes a sudden movement of the head or sits up suddenly.

ACTION — For otitis externa: Treatment consists of special drops prescribed by a physician, which often can be used just before and just after swimming to help prevent recurrences. If the canal is swollen shut, some temporary loss of hearing will be evident, but outer canal infections do not affect hearing on a permanent basis. Occasionally a spillover of infected material spreads infection from the middle ear; in this case, too, treatment consists of eardrops prescribed for the external component of the infection.

For otitis media: The doctor generally prescribes an antibiotic, not so much for the ear problem itself (which may be minimal and may clear up) but to avoid a more serious infection such as MASTOIDITIS or MENINGITIS. Once the acute symptoms of a middle ear infection have cleared, the child should be rechecked to make sure there is no fluid left in the cavity of the middle ear, which could thicken and interfere with the workings of the tiny bones there.

For otitis interna: Treatment depends on the severity of the infection and, of course, on whether it has spread from such a delicate site as the brain. Usually antibiotics and bed rest clear up an inner ear infection.

Parents should keep in mind that children's ear problems tend to recur. If you have eardrops previously prescribed for the same child within the past year, you may use them, but be sure to call the child's doctor if the problem persists. *Never* use an adult's prescription (such as an antibiotic) or another child's medication to treat a child who may have an ear infection. Even when the discomfort eases, the child should probably be examined by a doctor to make sure that the infection is not a complication of some more serious problem. Because of children's susceptibility to upper-respiratory infections, recurrences of ear problems can be expected. Parents should not be alarmed by these recurrences as long as each episode is promptly and properly treated.

See SWIMMER'S EAR

Eczema

A skin rash characterized by redness, itching, scaling, and crusting; in some cases, blistering may occur.

In children, eczema is usually related to an ALLERGY, and the youngster is apt to suffer other allergic reactions, such as ASTHMA.

In infants, the condition usually occurs between about six months and one year, with reddish-colored, crusty raised marks on the cheeks. Sometimes a parent notices cracks behind the child's ears. More often, lesions appear on the arms and legs, especially in the depressions in front of the elbows and behind the knees. Another form of the disorder generally occurs in children over the age of one. The lesions are raised and roundish, often filled with fluid, and intensely itchy.

The most serious form of eczema, called generalized eczema, is most often encountered in children over four years old. Almost the entire body is covered with running, crusty, itchy skin eruptions.

ACTION — The child's doctor may prescribe cortisone and a medicated lotion, and possibly a special diet that restricts milk intake. Parents can provide some relief from the itching by not bathing the child so often and by using cornstarch or bath oils in the bathwater as a means of decreasing skin dryness. It is wise to follow common-sense hygienic measures in efforts to avoid secondary bacterial infections of skin that is already ravaged by eczema.

Medical treatment is essential, not only for general supervision of treatment, which may include antihistamines and the use of corticosteroid compounds, but also for emotional counseling. Children may subconsciously use their eczema to exercise undue control over the family; also, stress tends to worsen the disease. This could lead to a vicious cycle of emotional instability for parents and the family in general.

Encephalitis

An inflammation of the brain.

Encephalitis is a fairly broad diagnostic term that also covers certain kinds of inflammations that are of noninfectious origins, for example, as a complication of other diseases, disorders, or diagnostic procedures. However, most commonly encephalitis is caused by a viral infection. The infection may be spread by virus-carrying insects or animals with rabies, or it may be a complication of viral diseases such as MEASLES, CHICKEN POX, INFLUENZA, MUMPS, and INFECTIOUS

MONONUCLEOSIS. Parents should be reassured that rarely do such common childhood illnesses lead to encephalitis, but it is a possibility.

Parents should also know that in the mosquito-carried St. Louis encephalitis, the leading cause of epidemic viral encephalitis in the United States, only 1 percent of all infections actually lead to symptoms — the other 99 percent show no symptoms and may actually acquire long-term immunity to the disease. In that 1 percent, the symptoms may vary, but a vast majority of those infected become gravely ill. However, it is less severe in children than adults; the death rate is 6 percent for all ages, but less than 1 percent in children under the age of five.

Aside from the symptom of stiff neck — which could also indicate MENINGITIS, with which encephalitis can be confused until appropriate diagnostic tests are performed — the first evidence of the disease is not very specific. Children may show fever, which may induce disordered thinking or even hallucinations; intensely severe headache; protracted, almost unrelenting vomiting; and lethargy that may progress to coma. Convulsions, temper outbursts, bizarre movements, hyperactivity, and loss of bowel and bladder control may occur.

ACTION — Encephalitis is extremely serious and demands prompt medical attention. Therefore, even if the disease's first signs and symptoms seem rather unspecific, parents should immediately seek medical help when children show the slightest evidence of possible encephalitis. Treatment is basically aimed at maintaining life and overcoming impaired functioning of vital organ systems such as the lungs and heart. If a BACTERIAL INFECTION is suspected, or at least until it is firmly excluded as a cause, physicians usually inject antibiotics as a precaution.

Compare MENINGITIS

Endocarditis

Inflammation of the membrane called the endocardium, *which lines the heart and its valves.*

Endocarditis usually occurs as a result of bacteria trapped around the heart valves. Before the advent of antibiotics, endocarditis was frequently one of the dangerous aftermaths of RHEUMATIC FEVER.

ACTION — Modern treatment consists of a prolonged course of antibiotics; bed rest is no longer considered necessary. Those children whose endocarditis is connected with heart-valve disease should also be given preventive antibiotic therapy whenever they need to undergo any surgery, such as dental extractions.

Enteritis

See GASTROENTERITIS, REGIONAL ENTERITIS

Epiglottitis

See CROUP

Epilepsy

See SEIZURE DISORDERS

Epstein-Barr Virus

See INFECTIOUS MONONUCLEOSIS

Eye, Lazy

See STRABISMUS

Eye Infections

Viral or bacterial insults of the eye.

At first the eye may appear red, with a clear, watery drainage. Itchiness usually causes the child to rub the eye, which aggravates the symptoms. As the infection becomes worse, the drainage becomes thickened and turns yellow-green. When the itching subsides, the child shows marked discomfort when exposed to a strong light and he or she complains, verbally or by crying, of considerable pain.

ACTION — Since the eye is such a sensitive and important organ, professional evaluation and treatment are necessary. Prescription antibiotic drops are usually given.

F

Fallen Arches

See FLAT FEET

Farsightedness

A visual disorder technically known as hyperopia *or* hypermetropia.

Farsightedness occurs when the eyeball is too short from front to back. As a result of this abnormality, light is focused slightly behind the retina and the child sees blurred images of objects that are close to the eye, while vision for faraway objects is not affected.

Most babies are somewhat farsighted at birth. As the eye grows during normal development, it usually allows the lens to focus images directly on the retina. Occasionally the shape of the eyeball continues to remain too short from front to back. For a time the lens can adjust by changing its shape so that rays of light are focused where they should be. But in order to accomplish this, the eye's ciliary muscles are under tension for long periods of time, which can cause eyestrain and eye discomfort until the condition is corrected.

ACTION — Parents should be sure their preschooler's eyes are examined, especially if signs of strain are evident. In less severe forms of farsightedness, corrective lenses may have to be worn only when the child is reading or doing other close work.

Fever Blister

See COLD SORE, HERPES SIMPLEX

Fever Convulsion

A brief episode of generalized seizure (involuntary muscle move-ments) brought on by fever. Loss of consciousness and jerking move-ments of the extremities and trunk are common and may be quite vigorous.

Fever convulsions occur in some 3 percent to 5 percent of otherwise healthy children, more often in boys than in girls. Although the convul-sions may be seen as late as ages 6 to 8, they usually occur between 6 months and 2 or 3 years of age, with a peak at around 18 months. Parents should be reassured that fever convulsions are not usually significant and appear to be something most children outgrow. They occur most commonly when there is a rapid and sudden temperature rise.

ACTION — Although there is generally no harm done by the seizure itself, the child should certainly be protected. If vomiting occurs, the parent should turn the child's head to one side and keep the airway clear. Be certain that breathing continues after the convulsion. The child should then be wrapped warmly and taken immediately to an emergency medical facility. After a first such seizure, a spinal tap may be taken if doctors suspect MENINGITIS, a disorder that also causes generalized convulsions.

Long-term management depends on the age of the child, the num-ber of times seizures have occurred, family history of fever seizures, and certain diagnostic tests such as the electroencephalogram (EEG), which measures brain waves.

Fifth Disease

A mild viral infection of childhood that features a sudden and typi-cal face rash with a "slapped cheek" appearance.

Fifth disease rash, which may also appear on the trunk and limbs, eventually fades into a pink, mottled, lacelike pattern, and there is usually little or no fever. After an incubation period of approximately one week, the illness may last up to ten days, with the rash persisting or recurring off and on for another two or three weeks.

The disease, known medically as *erythema infectiosum*, is called fifth disease because it is the fifth of five illnesses that produce some-what similar rashes. The other four illnesses are RUBELLA, MEASLES,

SCARLET FEVER, and a rare and mild form of scarlet fever called Filatov-Dukes disease.

ACTION — Complications are rare and no treatment is necessary. A child with fifth disease need not be isolated or kept from attending school. Since, however, an infection with the virus causing fifth disease may result in fetal death, pregnant women may not wish to have contact with a child who is infectious with the disease (a few days after the onset of the fever and rash). These recommendations are currently being reviewed.

Flat Feet

A condition in which one or both of the arches of the feet are flat.

It is normal for babies and small youngsters to have flat feet. The connective tissues in their feet are very soft and pliable. When these young children stand, it seems as though the arch flattens completely. However, when they sit, you can see a very definite curve to the bottom of the foot. As growth continues, the arch will strengthen regardless of whether shoes are worn. Parents should also know that the arch is variable from one child to another. Only about 15 percent of children have no arch at all, a condition generally called fallen arches.

ACTION — Except for a type of flat foot caused by a tight heel cord, in which stretching exercises may help, there is usually no treatment prescribed. Sometimes special shoes may provide more comfort, but the correction exists only when the shoes are worn. Pads sometimes used to build up an arch may produce discomfort.

Flu

See INFLUENZA

Food Poisoning

An acute illness caused by eating food that has been contaminated with pathogenic (disease-causing) bacteria or food that contains natural poisons, such as poisonous toadstools mistaken for harmless mushrooms.

The most common form of food poisoning is caused by eating food contaminated by *Salmonella*. These bacteria multiply in food that has been left in opened and unrefrigerated cans, in food that has been improperly canned or preserved, or in meats and other foods left too long in warmth or heat (an environment that favors rapid growth of bacteria).

The incubation period — the time from eating contaminated food to the onset of the first symptoms of the disease — is between 6 and 48 hours. Salmonellosis produces GASTROENTERITIS (inflammation of the lining of the stomach and intestines), usually causing diarrhea and vomiting and sometimes draining the body of enough fluids and essential mineral salts to create dehydration, a condition particularly harmful to infants. Sometimes the illness lasts only one or two days and may be so mild that bed rest and medical treatment are not required.

ACTION — The doctor should certainly be notified when children are first suspected of experiencing symptoms of food poisoning. BOTULISM, a much more serious form of food poisoning, may have to be considered. If possible, the doctor should be given a sample of the food that is suspected of having caused the illness. Fluids can usually be replaced by drinking solutions such as Pedialyte or Lytren. The liquid should be tepid and should be sipped very slowly, using a teaspoon if necessary, to prevent the recurrence of vomiting.

Fracture

A break in the normal structure of a bone or a tooth, usually the result of an injury.

Pain at the site of injury is a predominant symptom of a fracture. Parents may also note swelling and discoloration of the overlying tissues. At times a loss of contour is noticeable. Children may also experience numbness in an extremity, a pale demeanor, and, especially in infants and toddlers, fussiness and irritability. Any rapid discoloration farther out in the extremity from the site of injury may mean damage to a major blood vessel; emergency surgery may be necessary.

Occasionally fractures — especially of the collarbone — may occur at delivery. Collarbone fractures are also not uncommon in infants and toddlers, who may simply stop using the arm on the affected side and/or cry when the arm is moved. Special bandages can be applied to lessen the discomfort as healing takes place.

At times, seemingly minor acts such as jumping off a chair are sufficient to break a bone in the lower leg. And the falls common to childhood result fairly often in broken arms.

ACTION — When a fracture is suspected, restrict movement of the affected part and take the child to an emergency room or a physician's office. The doctor generally uses x-rays to confirm the nature of the fracture, then realigns the bone and immobilizes the affected part, usually in a cast. Parents should be sure they receive thorough instructions about cast care, especially if the child is too young to carry any of the responsibility.

Frostbite

Damage to the skin caused by exposure to extreme cold. Fingers, toes, ears, and nose are most commonly stricken.

Immediate treatment of frostbite consists of simply allowing the affected areas to rewarm slowly. Do *not* immerse in hot water, rub with snow, or attempt massage. Do *not*, as used to be recommended, immerse in cold water either.

ACTION — If sensation and normal coloring do not return within a short time, consult the child's doctor at once. Permanent damage or even gangrene (localized death of the affected tissues) can result if medical treatment is delayed.

Fungus Infections

See ATHLETE'S FOOT, DIAPER RASH, JOCK ITCH, RINGWORM, YEAST INFECTION

G

Gastroenteritis

Inflammation of the stomach and intestinal tract, especially the small intestine.

Gastroenteritis may be thought of as infectious diarrhea caused by viruses, bacteria, protozoa, fungi, or worms. When an exact infectious cause is determined, the signs and symptoms of the infection are given specific names, such as AMEBIC DYSENTERY or BACILLARY DYSENTERY. Sometimes FOOD POISONING or taking toxic chemicals can cause gastroenteritis; various tropical diseases can also play a role.

Viral gastroenteritis tends to be rather mild and usually clears up in a few days. Bacterial gastroenteritis is more serious. It is marked by the sudden development of severe diarrhea, which sometimes may be bloody. Vomiting and fever are typical; delirium and symptoms of shock from poisoning are less common, but they may occur.

ACTION — Any type of gastroenteritis can be extremely dangerous to infants because of the chance of dehydration, which can occur very quickly, although the time can vary from child to child. Hospitalization — so that fluids can be replaced intravenously and the child can be monitored — is generally necessary. In fact, any child who has lost more than 10 percent of his or her weight because of fluid loss should probably be hospitalized.

Less severe dehydration can be treated at home by restricting solids and milk and placing the child on a clear liquid diet until the condition clears and the doctor approves a gradual reintroduction of solid foods. Parents should understand that a liquid diet means *lots* of liquids. Children need around 4½ ounces of fluid for each 2¼ pounds of body weight. A 30-pound child therefore requires more than 2 quarts of clear fluid each day. This diet can be varied by using weakened tea, different fruit juices, water, and even carbonated beverages if the

71

child's doctor approves. The ideal replacement is one of the commercially balanced electrolyte solutions available at most pharmacies.

Parents should keep in mind that antispasmodics, antidiarrheal medicines, and preparations that stop vomiting may mask symptoms of dehydration. These medicines should never be given to infants and small children unless a physician is carefully supervising the youngsters.

German Measles

See RUBELLA

Gilles de la Tourette's Syndrome

See TOURETTE'S SYNDROME

Growing Pains

Limb pain peculiar to growing children.

Once ascribed to children's vivid imaginations, it is now thought that these joint and muscle pains are probably related to the growth and changing composition of muscles. Some children experience marked discomfort in the arms or legs with normal play, although the pain is heightened by strenuous exercise such as engaging in sports. Rest, warm baths, the application of heat, and the use of mild painkillers such as children's doses of aspirin usually offer some relief.

ACTION — If there is no joint swelling, no fever, no muscle weakness, and no weight loss, a doctor's care is probably not needed.

H

Hay Fever

Seasonal ALLERGY *that strikes in spring and summer, when airborne pollen is prevalent.*

The name hay fever is misleading: Fever does not occur, and the signs and symptoms result from sensitivity to many wind-borne pollens from trees, grasses, and weeds. Hay fever, also known by the medical term *allergic rhinitis*, can be caused by exposure to indoor allergens that are inhaled, such as house dust, feathers, and animal hair.

The symptoms and signs of hay fever can occur suddenly or develop gradually. An early indication may be intense itching of the nose, throat, and roof of the mouth. This is followed or accompanied by sneezing, watering of the eyes (which sometimes become red and itchy), and a discharge of clear thin fluid from the nose. Nasal congestion, when the lining of the nose swells, makes breathing difficult. When the pollen count is particularly high, the air tubes of the lungs may be involved, so that the child has brief, asthmalike attacks with wheezing.

ACTION — Children who suffer badly from hay fever should see a doctor. When a specific type of pollen is identified as the allergen, it may be possible to desensitize the child through a series of injections that stimulate the body to produce an immune response. This treatment should be begun at least three to four months before the start of the hay fever season. This kind of treatment is undertaken, however, only if the symptoms are severe.

Milder forms of hay fever can often be dramatically relieved by taking antihistamines. Some of these drugs are available over the counter, but more potent ones can be obtained with a doctor's prescription. Parents should be sure — as with all drugs given to children — that label instructions are followed carefully.

Heart Murmurs

Abnormal sounds heard by a physician listening to the heart with a stethoscope.

Functional murmurs — absolutely harmless ones — are quite common in children. They are caused by turbulence in the blood as it flows through the heart. Approximately 15 percent to 20 percent of the population has such murmurs, and they live full and active lives without the need for any medical or surgical treatment to correct the murmur. Functional murmurs do not lead to heart disease, and many of them go away spontaneously as the child gets older.

Even organic murmurs — those that may signify some defect in the heart or its valves — do not generally cause any limitation of activity.

ACTION — Regularly scheduled physical examinations permit the doctor to monitor the situation and detect problems before they become major. Sometimes antibiotics are prescribed to prevent infections should any operations or major dental procedures be done.

In addition to the physician's physical examination, several diagnostic tests are used to investigate the heart. The electrocardiogram (EKG) makes a tracing of heart activity. Chest x-rays indicate whether the heart may be enlarged. The echocardiogram uses sound waves to depict the way the heart is working. In cardiac catheterization, a dye is injected so that specialists can actually see how the heart is functioning. The results of these tests help the doctor prescribe the correct course of treatment.

Heartburn

See INDIGESTION

Heat Rash

A skin inflammation in which pinpoint blisters progress to a bright red, dotted appearance.

In severe cases of heat rash — technically known as *miliaria* and also called *prickly heat* — the spots seem to join into one large rash. Heat rash occurs when excessive heat or too-heavy clothing causes a blockage of the sweat glands. Infants are particularly prone to heat rash because of the immaturity of their skin structure. The cheeks, neck, trunk, and diaper areas are commonly involved.

ACTION — The condition is not harmful, and there is no specific treatment. Parents should avoid overdressing babies when the weather is hot. Cool baths and the application of a light medicated powder may reduce the irritation, and the child may be more comfortable in an air-conditioned or air-cooled environment. Prevention of prickly heat involves avoiding high temperatures and humidity, keeping out of direct sunlight, and dressing in porous, nonbinding clothes.

Heat Stroke and Heat Exhaustion

An acute illness resulting from prolonged exposure to high environmental temperatures.

Heat exhaustion or heat stroke happens like this: In an attempt to maintain normal body temperature, the child sweats excessively, causing a loss of body fluids and salts. The child appears pale, and the skin is cold and clammy. Beads of perspiration may appear on the forehead. Shallow breathing is usually present, and sometimes the child vomits or feels like vomiting. Confusion is a late sign. Left unattended, the child lapses into unconsciousness.

ACTION — As soon as the situation is discovered, remove the child to a cool place. Place the youngster on his or her back with the head lowered and the feet elevated. Cover the child with a blanket and phone an emergency medical unit for help. If conscious, children with heat stroke may be given short sips of saltwater (one teaspoonful of salt to one pint of water).

Compare SUNSTROKE

Hemangioma

Small benign (not malignant) tumors that are among the most common congenital (present-at-birth) defects seen in children. They may occur in any organ of the body, but they are usually found on the skin.

Hemangiomas affect the vascular system and appear as a disorganized collection of small blood vessels, usually in a well-circumscribed area. By far the most common of the hemangiomas is the "salmon patch." This irregular, reddened, flat area on the forehead or the upper eyelids appears in up to 40 percent of all newborn babies. Many infants also have similar marks on the back of the scalp and the nape of the neck. The overwhelming majority of these marks spontaneously disappear by the time the child is one; no treatment is necessary. Occasionally the patches are noticeable later in life whenever the child cries or is flushed, but there is no real disfigurement.

The "strawberry hemangioma" is a raised, red-to-purple mass that develops during the first few months of life; it may be noticeable at birth. It starts out as a tiny red spot anywhere on the body, but usually on the face, neck, or trunk. Over the first six months of life, the strawberry mark enlarges rapidly; most of them reach their final size by the time the child is one year old. Some "strawberries" may reach two to three inches across, raised from one-half to one inch from the skin, before they stop growing. Then, for several months, the size may remain stable. But as the mass outgrows its own blood supply, it begins to whiten and shrink in size. Most of these hemangiomas are gone by the time the child is three years old; all that remains is a faint discoloration of the skin or, in some cases, no mark at all. Very large hemangiomas, for example, those that may cover an entire half of the child's face, may take longer to go away.

The "cavernous hemangioma" is a tangled mass of blood vessels; it tends to lie deeper in the skin. The tumor has an irregular border and a soft, bubbly consistency. Many are noticed at birth, but some will not become evident until the baby is a few months old. Sometimes a purplish discoloration is all that is seen; sometimes the mass sticks up from the skin's surface. They grow more slowly than strawberry hemangiomas, and they take longer to go away if, indeed, they do go away.

"Port wine stains" are pink-to-red flat marks that usually occur on the face. They vary in size and have irregular borders. Port wine stains grow as the child grows and, unlike strawberry marks and cavernous hemangiomas, they do not go away spontaneously. In the past, treatment has not been very satisfactory, but with current treatment excellent results can be obtained.

ACTION — For strawberry hemangiomas: Ordinarily no treatment is required, and parents can rest assured that their child is not disfigured for life. Only if a vital organ such as the eye is involved need special medical attention be undertaken. Occasionally the center of the hemangioma will ooze and crust as it breaks down. If that happens, infection could set in, and an antibiotic cream may be needed.

For cavernous hemangiomas: Because of their depth, there is usually no disfiguration and no treatment is needed unless some vital organ is affected.

For port wine stains: Currently, therapy that involves use of an argon laser beam is showing some promising results. The procedure lightens the port wine stain considerably, but it is not recommended for children younger than nine. A few cosmetic companies have devised bases and coverups that make the mark much less noticeable.

Hemophilia

An inherited disease in which the blood fails to clot within the time range generally considered normal, which can result in severe and life-threatening bleeding.

Hemophilia is a genetic disease that affects males, but the defect is carried by females who are generally symptomless. The defect involves abnormalities in the blood-clotting factor, which can be diagnosed by laboratory tests that reveal functional defects and a lowered quantity of clotting factor. A carrier has about a 50-50 chance of passing the genetic defect to her daughters, who will themselves be carriers with an equal chance of passing on the defect. A male hemophiliac cannot pass on the disease to his sons, but all his daughters will be carriers, since the disease is sex-linked to the X chromosome in body cells.

The disorder may be noticed very early, for example, with excessive bleeding at circumcision; in milder forms, it may not become evident until the boy has a tooth extracted or has minor surgery. Often a minor scrape or cut causes abnormal bleeding, and the hemophiliac may show large and deep-seated bruises as a result of extremely minor burns or injuries that other children incur almost daily without difficulty.

Hemophilia is rare. It is estimated that there are approximately 25,000 hemophiliacs in the United States — which means an incidence of only about 1 in 10,000. However, without parental understanding of what the disease means and without appropriate treatment, boys with hemophilia can literally bleed to death or develop crippling deformities from blood seeping into body joints.

ACTION — The disease can be managed by infusion of a substance called cryoprecipitate. This material is prepared by adding the clotting factor to plasma that is quick-frozen, then slow-thawed. Parents can actively participate in their child's therapy by learning how to infuse cryoprecipitate at home. Should bleeding occur at an easily accessible body area, applying direct hand pressure or elastic bandages can usually control the bleeding until the child reaches the doctor's office or an emergency medical facility. Other drugs may be prescribed that will lessen bleeding in the case of dental extraction or minor surgery.

Counseling may be of great benefit. Both the parents and the affected child need support in their efforts to maintain as normal a lifestyle as possible. Also, some parents may want to review their plans to have additional children in light of the risk of transmitting hemophilia.

Hepatitis

Inflammation of the liver, most commonly caused by a VIRAL INFECTION.

Infectious hepatitis was once thought to be transmitted solely by drinking or eating food contaminated with infected human feces where, for example, poor sewage facilities existed. Serum hepatitis was thought to be transmitted solely by using contaminated blood in transfusions or through injections with contaminated needles or syringes. It is now known that both forms of viral hepatitis, now called hepatitis A (infectious) and hepatitis B (serum), can be transmitted by either route, though one generally predominates.

Hepatitis A, also known as short-term hepatitis, is the more common form in children. It is most often transmitted by the feces-to-mouth route, but the disease is highly contagious. The incubation period is generally from two to seven weeks. Children may become listless or cranky.

Hepatitis B, also called long-incubation hepatitis, is potentially the more serious form of viral hepatitis. It is generally spread through blood and blood products, or from the mother to the fetus. It is also transmitted through intimate contact, such as sexual intercourse, and from drug user to drug user via shared needles. Hospital instruments tainted by the hepatitis B virus are often resistant to standard sterilization techniques. The incubation period for hepatitis B may be 7 to 26 weeks from exposure to infection.

Early symptoms of hepatitis B often resemble those of influenza. The urine may appear dark, and the stools frequently take on a grayish color. Other indications typically include a general feeling of malaise (a vague sense of being unwell), fever, and later development of JAUNDICE. However, jaundice may not appear, especially in those who have had a previous infection and have developed at least partial immunity. The child usually has no appetite and is apt to become weak and drowsy.

Mild forms of hepatitis are often associated with and seem to be a result of the Epstein-Barr virus.

ACTION — For hepatitis A: If the child has been around a hepatitis patient, parents should contact a doctor and inquire about the advisability of gamma globulin injections as a preventive measure. Home treatment, mostly consisting of bed rest and/or restriction of activity, is usually possible. Because of the contagiousness of the disease, other family members and close contacts should be given preventive injections of gamma globulin.

For hepatitis B: Children with hepatitis B need strict bed rest. In severe cases, hospitalization may be needed, especially if intravenous solutions of glucose (sugar) are needed to compensate for dehydration. Steroids used to control the disease are essentially useless and may increase the chances of liver damage. But much hope has been invested in the use of the prescription drug alpha interferon, especially in conjunction with steroids.

Once the child has hepatitis, no specific drug therapy is effective. However, the outlook for full recovery is very favorable. Even a severely damaged liver has a remarkable capacity for regeneration.

More information may be obtained by calling the American Liver Foundation toll-free at 800-223-0179, Monday through Friday, 8:30 A.M. to 4:30 P.M. eastern time (201-256-2550 in New Jersey).

See also AIDS, INFECTIOUS MONONUCLEOSIS

Hernia

A piece of body tissue that has ruptured through an opening and is sticking out from whatever structure normally confines it.

A hernia may occur at any site in the body, as, for example, a herniated vertebral disc (a slipped disc). Children most often suffer from umbilical hernias or inguinal (groin) hernias. An umbilical hernia is a bulge beneath the area where the umbilical cord was attached.

Sometimes while the baby is still in the uterus, cord tissues fail to close. Umbilical hernias are more common in girls than in boys and occur in black children more so than in whites.

Although occasionally an infant will have a bulge as large as an orange, most umbilical hernias are small, becoming more noticeable when the baby cries. There is no pain. The bulge usually consists of intestine and supporting structures that protrude through the opening in the abdominal wall. This is, of course, all inside. What you see on the baby's abdomen is simply a skin-covered bulge that tends to recede under slight pressure.

Inguinal hernias may appear at any time of life. Most often a portion of the intestinal tract slides in and out of the scrotum in males. Less commonly, intestinal material protrudes directly through the abdominal wall into the groin area — a defect that can be seen in girls as well as boys. Like umbilical hernias, they usually arise because certain tissues did not close properly when the fetus was developing; an opening remains through which the intestine bulges out.

When inguinal hernias are seen in boys, parents may note a bulge alongside the penis or in the scrotum itself. In girls, the mass appears in the groin area alongside the external genitals.

A particular problem is incarceration; that is, when the hernia slides, it gets locked in and is unable to move. Pain, irritability, problems with bowel movements, and pressure may develop.

On rare occasions, an infant will be born with a diaphragmatic hernia, in which the abdominal contents poke through an abnormal opening that exists in the diaphragm, the large muscle sheet that separates the abdominal and chest spaces. The baby will have trouble breathing, and immediate surgery must be performed. In other instances, when the defect is very small, it takes days for trouble to occur.

ACTION — For umbilical hernias: Some controversy lingers about the usefulness of strapping with "belly binders," but it is generally thought that these measures do not help and may possibly do harm. No treatment is required; most umbilical hernias recede by themselves by the time the child is one or two, although it may take until about age five if the bulge is unusually large. Surgery should be avoided unless complications, such as pain or intestinal blockage, occur.

For inguinal hernias: If swelling in the loop of bowel occurs, an INTESTINAL OBSTRUCTION will develop, and the hernia is said to be

strangulated. Emergency surgery is necessary. Otherwise, an inguinal hernia can normally wait for elective surgery, at a time when the
child is older and surgical risks are diminished. Parents should bear
in mind, however, that if any bulge is hard, if pain is present, or if
symptoms such as vomiting and abdominal bloating are present,
emergency medical treatment should be sought immediately.

For diaphragmatic hernias: The infant is treated with various
emergency procedures to assist breathing before and after surgery.

Herpangina

*A viral illness characterized by small ulcers in the mouth and on the
gums, with fevers as high as 105° F.*

The infection lasts for three or four days and then goes away by
itself.

ACTION — No active treatment is necessary, but the parent can offer
the child some relief by giving cool liquids, a fever-reducer such as
aspirin, and perhaps by dabbing the sores with a cotton swab dipped
in an astringent mouthwash. Parents should also watch for any sign
of dehydration if the infant or child absolutely refuses to drink.

Herpes Simplex

An infectious disease caused by a virus of the same name.

Herpes simplex is often referred to merely as herpes, but it should
not be confused with the totally separate disease known as HERPES
ZOSTER, commonly known as shingles, or with herpes virus Type II,
which causes genital infections in adults.

The disorder is marked by the formation of groups of small cold
sores or fever blisters at the corners of the mouth, around the eyes
(ocular herpes), on the genitals (herpes genitalis), or occasionally on
other parts of the body.

Even though a baby will not have Type II herpes, infants born to
women with a genital herpes infection may suffer neonatal herpes by
becoming infected during passage through the birth canal. This, in
turn, can lead to meningoencephalitis (a dangerous inflammation of
the child's brain and membranes that cover the brain). To avoid this
situation, women with genital herpes are usually advised to give birth
by cesarean section.

ACTION — For affected children, no specific treatment exists, although special antiviral creams have recently been developed that may help control the severity and extent of the lesions.

Herpes Zoster

A viral disease in which the roots of sensory nerves just outside the spinal cord are affected.

This leads to a red rash and blisters, generally occurring on only one side of the body — for example, one side of the face, one shoulder or arm, or along one side of the chest or abdomen.

Herpes zoster, commonly known as shingles, is rare in children, although it sometimes occurs when the chicken pox virus, lying dormant since an episode of that common disease of childhood, is reactivated. The disease is usually mild in children, and the outlook for full recovery is very good.

ACTION — No specific treatment exists, although children may be given childhood doses of aspirin or acetaminophen for relief of pain if that becomes a problem.

Herpetic Stomatitis

Acute inflammation and blistering inside the mouth caused by the herpes virus.

The child may run a temperature as high as 104° or 105° F for a week to ten days. Intense mouth discomfort may cause a child to refuse to eat, and irritability is common. Although this infection is caused by a herpes virus, it is not the same one as is transmitted sexually.

ACTION — The disease clears up by itself, without complications, and no treatment is necessary. Applying cotton swabs dipped in an astringent mouthwash may offer some relief, as will cool liquids and aspirin or aspirinlike fever reducers given in children's doses.

Hiccups

A forceful body reflex resulting from a spasm of the diaphragm, the thin muscle sheet that separates the abdominal and chest cavities.

The sound made is characteristic, and from it comes the name. Hiccups tend to occur when the diaphragm or the nerves that supply it are subjected to pressure or irritation.

Infants often swallow air with feedings, which causes the stomach to increase in size, squeezing the diaphragm. Vigorous sucking and overfeeding make the problem worse. Frequent burping can help keep the stomach from distending too much. Older children may get hiccups from eating too rapidly or swallowing large quantities of carbonated beverages.

More serious medical conditions may be responsible, such as infections of the abdominal cavity, kidney failure, or a perforated ulcer. But if such a process is under way, there will be other symptoms far more dramatic than hiccups.

ACTION — In most instances of ordinary hiccups, no treatment is required. Many home remedies (drinking water with the head held forward and down, raising one's arms and holding one's breath) exist. But scaring a child is definitely not recommended. Only in the rarest of instances does prolonged hiccuping, which can become quite exhausting, necessitate medical attention.

Hip Dislocation

Improper joining of the hip.

Some babies are born with an abnormally lax hip joint — that is, it is abnormally mobile — and the knobby portion of bone slides easily in and out of its socket. In some instances, a dislocation can accidentally be caused during breech birth.

In most cases, this difficulty is spotted within a few days of birth and treatment, often with a splint or a specially padded diaper, is started immediately.

Hips that are not properly joined at birth are likely to become progressively less stable as the child grows. Hip joints weak at birth may not become truly dislocated for several months.

ACTION — Parents may be able to recognize the condition if one of the baby's legs seems slightly shorter than the other, or if unusual wrinkling of the skin exists on one of the child's thighs or buttocks. It is important to bring this to the attention of a physician, because the sooner a hip dislocation is noted, the easier it can be treated medically, without recourse to surgery.

Hives

A skin reaction, known by the medical name of urticaria, *that shows localized swellings or elevations of the skin that are red and intensely itchy.*

Occasionally hives are associated with viral infections (especially in younger children) or urinary-tract infections and STREP THROAT. However, by far the most common cause is ALLERGY. Hypersensitivity to a wide variety of substances causes histamine to "pour out" within the body, resulting in an accumulation of fluid in the skin or mucous membranes. Therefore, doctors generally prescribe antihistamines, although other approaches (special inhalants or medicines that thin mucus accumulations) are sometimes used.

ACTION — Cold compresses may offer some relief. If an underlying infection is present, it must be treated with antibiotics.

Hodgkin's Disease

A disorder in which there is a painless overgrowth of lymphatic glands throughout the body; red blood corpuscles are reduced in number, so that severe ANEMIA *develops; internal organs such as the spleen become enlarged.*

Although Hodgkin's disease often strikes in young adulthood, it also affects children — boys more often than girls. It is sometimes confused with LEUKEMIA; in fact, one of its technical names is *pseudoleukemia*. However, it appears not to be neoplastic (a true cancer), and it is not marked by the overwhelming increase in white blood cells found in leukemia.

Lymphatic enlargement may occur first in the neck, then the armpits and the groin, and finally inside the deep internal glands and organs. There is little if any pain, but fever, HERPES ZOSTER, a bronze discoloration of the skin, and profound weakness are common.

ACTION — Aggressive medical treatment with modern drugs or x-ray therapy — undertaken by a certified oncologist or hematologist/ oncologist, preferably at a university hospital — offers some relief from symptoms, and remissions of several years are not uncommon. However, the disease remains a very serious one for which no permanent cure is yet known. Therefore, family counseling may help the parents, siblings, and the sufferer come to terms with this illness.

Compare LEUKEMIA

Hole in the Heart

A congenital (present-at-birth) malformation in which a septal defect permits abnormal flow of blood from one heart chamber to another.

The two upper heart chambers, called atria, are separated by a membranous wall called the atrial septum. Incomplete development allows an atrial septal defect or hole. The thick and muscular bottom chambers that pump blood out into the body, called ventricles, are separated by another septum. Incomplete development here creates a ventricular septal defect or hole.

Because a hole in the heart disrupts the normal passage of blood into and out of the heart, the baby does not get enough oxygen circulating and may look bluish in color. Diagnosis, now frequently made soon after birth, depends on physical findings, chest x-rays, heart tracings done by electrocardiograph, and, if indicated, a heart catheterization. The latter test involves the injection of a dye directly into the bloodstream while special heart x-rays are taken.

ACTION — Treatment, either medical or surgical, depends on the degree of symptoms and the extent of the heart abnormality. Parents should be reassured that current medical practice allows increasingly successful treatment with minimal or no remaining disability.

Hydrocele

A collection of fluid around a testicle or the cord to the testicle.

This is not uncommon in newborns, in whom the scrotal sac on the affected side appears swollen and tense. It can also be diagnosed by simply passing light from a flashlight through the scrotum.

ACTION — The fluid will be absorbed by the body and the swelling will disappear, usually within the first year of life. There is no adverse effect and no treatment is necessary. However, hydroceles that develop later in infancy or after the baby is one year old should be managed differently because of the possibility of an associated HERNIA, for which surgery might be indicated.

Hypercholesteremia

Too high a level of cholesterol in the blood.

Cholesterol is a waxy substance found in food as well as produced by the body; most of the body's cholesterol is made by the body, but some comes from a diet containing animal fats such as milk, eggs, and meat. Cholesterol is needed by the body for hormone production and to form the myelin sheaths around nerve fibers.

When the body produces more cholesterol than it needs, or does not eliminate it well enough, or when the diet is heavy in saturated fats, which can elevate the cholesterol level in the blood, then the stage is set for development of certain diseases, including gallstones, hardening of the arteries, and some cancers. Genetics plays a part in certain people's tendency to have hypercholesteremia.

Although children rarely exhibit these negative effects of excessive cholesterol, it is commonly held that high serum cholesterol levels in children are signs of the beginning of hardened plaques forming on blood vessel walls, which over the course of years may narrow the passage for the flow of blood and lead to coronary artery disease and possibly heart attacks. Autopsies on young accident victims have shown that fatty deposits have already begun to form on their coronary arteries.

The current thinking is that the level of cholesterol in a child's blood will increase as he or she grows up, so it can be very important for parents to help their offspring maintain an adequately low level in childhood so that the inevitable rise will not produce high levels associated with health risks. Cholesterol readings of 160 to 180 milligrams per deciliter (mg/dl) are considered in the healthy range for adults, and some evidence suggests that a child would need to have a reading of about 140 to 160 mg/dl to remain in the healthy range upon reaching maturity. To remain in the safe range — which, in adults, is under 200 mg/dl — a child's reading would need to be not much higher than 170 mg/dl.

Yet some recent studies seem to suggest that perhaps commonly held beliefs have been wrong — that there is little correlation between the cholesterol levels one has as a child and the ultimate cholesterol level attained as an adult, and that putting children on cholesterol-lowering diets will not reduce the risk of heart disease later on in life. These are, not surprisingly, controversial findings in what is a fairly controversial field of study. Parents should stay alert to news and views about cholesterol, but avoid changing life-styles and attitudes with every new study or news story.

High cholesterol is something to be aware of and to have tracked, especially if parents and grandparents have the problem too. But parents should not go overboard in their attempts to eradicate what has been made by the media to appear to be public health enemy number one. Hypercholesteremia should be controlled, but it is only one of many risk factors that can add up to heartbreak — and heart disease — for your child when he or she grows up.

ACTION — It would seem prudent for parents to consider the type and content of food they give their children, especially if either or both of the parents have a familial history of heart disease. Although it may not be immediately critical to make a special trip to the physician for a blood test to check cholesterol levels, it can and perhaps should be done at the next regular checkup. If the total serum cholesterol reading is high, or the ratio between high-density lipoproteins (the so-called good cholesterol) and low-density lipoproteins (the so-called bad cholesterol) is low, then an adjustment in dietary fats is probably warranted for any child over the age of two years — an overzealous dietary fat restriction imposed on children under two years could lead to growth deficits. Increased exercise, weight loss (if necessary), and even seeking a professional to help with stress reduction for the child and the entire family are also avenues of action. Get guidance, food charts and recipes, and support from your doctor or health-care professional, a registered dietician, or a nutritionist. Dietary change need not be painful; it is easy enough to do at home, and restaurants all over the country provide heart-healthy and good-tasting items on their menus. It is extremely rare for a child to have cholesterol levels high enough to require any sort of drug intervention.

Hypermetropia

See FARSIGHTEDNESS

Hyperopia

See FARSIGHTEDNESS

Hypertension

Abnormally high blood pressure.

Hypertension is not common in children in the absence of some medical disorder that can be diagnosed and treated. However, recent studies have shown an undeniable link between high blood pressure and lack of physical fitness in children as young as five and six years of age; and the less fit and flabbier the child, the higher both the systolic and diastolic blood pressures are. Further, this link follows the child into adulthood, and can be a precursor of future cardiovascular health.

ACTION — Parents are urged to seek medical advice if their child is determined, for example, by a school nurse, to have high blood pressure. They should also get involved in making sure their children are physically active and eating balanced diets.

Compare HYPOTENSION

Hyperthyroidism

See THYROID DISORDERS

Hyperventilation

Breathing too fast and too much.

Children who are hyperventilating may also feel numbness or tingling sensations, a certain amount of weakness, or even faintness. Severe episodes may lead to muscle spasms and loss of consciousness, as the body is out of sync because an abnormal amount of carbon dioxide is being breathed out.

Occasionally hyperventilation indicates the presence of some disease, but more often than not it results from anxiety. Once a doctor has determined that there is no disease, children can often be helped merely by understanding that anxiety causes their symptoms and that they can avoid the symptoms by avoiding the anxiety. If this does not work, seek some professional counseling.

ACTION — The old paper bag trick actually works to treat hyperventilation. Get a paper bag large enough to cover the child's mouth and nose. Hold it very close to the child's face and have him or her breathe into the bag and rebreathe the air in the bag. If the child does this long enough, perhaps several tries of ten times in and ten times out between brief rests, the normal level of carbon dioxide in the bloodstream returns and the symptoms go away.

Medicines should not be used without approval of the child's doctor or health-care professional.

Hypoglycemia

An abnormally low level of glucose (sugar) in the circulating blood.

Symptoms of hypoglycemia include nervousness, cold sweats, weakness, a feeling of acute fatigue, irritability, and, in severe and untreated cases, mental disturbances such as confusion, hallucinations, or bizarre behavior. In extreme cases, particularly in a child with DIABETES MELLITUS, untreated hypoglycemia may result in loss of consciousness or even death.

Hypoglycemia is fairly common in newborn infants; approximately 4 out of every 1,000 full-term babies and about 16 out of every 1,000 premature babies have this condition. Prompt medical evaluation and treatment are usually successful in correcting the abnormality.

ACTION — Children with mild episodes respond to orange juice, honey, or other sweet substances. In moderate spells, a child also needs carbohydrates that can be absorbed more slowly, such as a banana, apple, bread, or cereals. Children with severe reactions should always be taken to a doctor for evaluation and for more sophisticated care, such as administration of glucagon.

Hypotension

Abnormally low blood pressure.

Hypotension is even more rare in children than HYPERTENSION — it is so rare, in fact, that most references fail to list specific guidelines — occurring mostly in the instance of severe SHOCK.

ACTION — If a child is found to have blood pressure readings lower than average, he or she should be checked by a physician or appropriate health-care professional.

Hypothermia

A condition in which the body's temperature drops below its norm.

Hypothermia is very rare in infants and children unless they are subjected to extreme deprivation (e.g., lack of heat and warm clothing) or, for example, they are exposed to freezing temperatures over a prolonged period of time. In extreme cases, the body's temperature may drop dramatically and prove fatal.

ACTION — In very sick or premature infants, in whom the body's metabolic needs create rapid heat loss, isolette (incubator) temperatures may have to be regulated by hospital staff in order to encourage maintenance of the baby's normal body temperature.

Hypothyroidism

See THYROID DISORDERS

I

Impetigo

A skin infection, technically called pyoderma, *caused when bacteria, usually* Staphylococci, *enter small breaks in the skin, such as those caused by insect bites or scratching.*

Impetigo may start as a small area of redness, generally with a blister. It spreads by scratching or simply because of the large number of staph bacteria present, which may invade other tiny skin breaks. The blisters ooze a yellow fluid that dries to form crusts.

Generally speaking, impetigo can be cured in a few days if treatment is applied vigorously as soon as the condition is noticed. If the sores do not stop spreading in three days, or if the child develops an oral temperature over 100° F, parents should consult a doctor for advice. If red streaks or localized swollen glands appear, the child should be taken to his or her doctor. Such signs may mean that the infection is burrowing deeper into tissues, causing an inflammation that may be heralded by redness, swelling, and pain.

Normally, complications do not occur, and parents can be reassured that the unsightly sores of impetigo do not leave permanent scars.

ACTION — The child should be bathed with an antibacterial soap, with each sore cleansed carefully. Crusts should be scraped away (soaking in warm water may ease removal), and an antibiotic ointment should be rubbed into the base of the sores. Some doctors prefer that the child also be given oral antibiotics to prevent complications and hasten healing.

Because impetigo is contagious, special hygienic measures must be observed by each member of the family, with special attention to separating the affected child's towels, bed linens, and clothes for special washing.

Indigestion

Imperfect or incomplete digestion, occasionally associated with a disease or some disorder of the digestive system, but most commonly caused by bad eating and drinking habits.

Children should be taught to chew their food slowly and thoroughly, to avoid excitement and strenuous exercise before and immediately after mealtimes, and to be careful not to swallow air while eating or drinking.

Eating gas-forming foods such as cabbage or beans or a lot of fried and fatty foods that may be undercooked can also contribute to indigestion. When the child eats the wrong kinds of food or too much food, the stomach and intestines can become distended (overstretched), which interferes with the natural wavelike motions that carry contents through the digestive tract and eliminate waste materials.

Heartburn is one symptom of indigestion. It has nothing at all to do with the heart but is a burning sensation in the chest caused by some of the stomach's acid contents flowing upward and into the lower part of the esophagus and irritating its delicate lining.

ACTION — Some relief of simple stomach upset can be obtained by taking one of the many nonprescription antacids. Label instructions for children's doses — if, indeed, the medicine is designed for children to take — should be followed carefully; it is even better for parents to call a physician or health-care professional for advice. The child should *not* be given aspirin or laxatives, because it is not always possible to be sure the discomfort is only indigestion.

Infantile Paralysis

See POLIOMYELITIS

Infectious Mononucleosis

An acute infectious disease caused by the Epstein-Barr (E-B) virus.

Commonly referred to simply as "mono," it can occur at any age, but it is especially prevalent in young adults, adolescents, and older children, particularly when large groups of young people live in close contact, such as at schools or camps.

The incubation period varies from four to about ten weeks. It is not clear how the infection is transmitted; kissing has often been implicated, but it is not a major mode of spread.

It starts gradually, and the symptoms are often mild. There is usually a sore throat; swollen glands, especially lymph glands in the neck, armpits, and groin; fatigue; and fever. In a few cases, a skin rash rather like that of RUBELLA (German measles) develops and, in even rarer cases, the young person may become jaundiced (yellowish). The virus frequently causes the liver and spleen to become inflamed. In most cases, symptoms subside within a few weeks, although fatigue and malaise (a general sense of being unwell) may persist for several weeks. Sometimes depression and general debility may linger after an unusually severe attack.

Diagnosis is made by a laboratory examination of a blood sample. The disorder causes an increase in certain types of white blood cells called lymphocytes and monocytes, and it may alter their appearance.

Parents need not worry unless serious complications arise. In that case, prompt medical attention should be sought. These signs, symptoms, and disorders include convulsions, HEPATITIS, ENCEPHALITIS, severe abdominal discomfort that might suggest a ruptured spleen, neck stiffness, PNEUMONIA, and any severe swelling of the tonsils or throat, which could cause serious breathing difficulties.

ACTION — No specific treatment is required, although bed rest is advised as long as the young person has a fever. Some physicians may prescribe a hormone called an adrenal corticosteroid, although certain other conditions may contraindicate this, and once prescribed, it should not be prescribed for any other illness during the next 12 months. The antibiotic ampicillin should not be given, because in about 80 percent of mono patients it can cause a skin rash. If a physician determines that the spleen is enlarged, contact sports and other vigorous activities must be stopped until healing has occurred.

Influenza

An acute and highly contagious VIRAL INFECTION *commonly known as the flu.*

The incubation period for influenza varies from about 24 to 48 hours. Symptoms appear suddenly: severe HEADACHE; aches in muscles and joints, especially BACKACHE; loss of appetite; sweating; and severe fatigue. Body temperature rises sharply to about 101° to 103° F (38° to 39.5° C). Generally, the fever and pain gradually subside within two or three days. Even though high fevers may persist for four or five days in a child with influenza, it is advisable to check with the child's doctor if a temperature over 101° or 102° F has been present for more than 24 hours.

Even when the temperature returns to normal, children often feel weak and slightly dizzy for a few days. A dry, hacking cough may persist for as long as a week or so after the other symptoms have disappeared. However, potentially serious complications from influenza are uncommon in children who are otherwise healthy.

In infants and younger children, the signs and symptoms are often similar to those resulting from other viral infections of the respiratory system. Some children experience FEVER CONVULSION, vomiting, diarrhea, otitis media (middle EAR INFECTION), high fever, clear nasal discharge, and fleeting skin rash.

ACTION — Drugs have no direct effect on the influenza virus, although the antivirus drug amantadine hydrochloride may minimize severity and duration if it is given early on. Other drugs, including antibiotics, may be given to treat a bacterial infection, such as PNEUMONIA.

Otherwise, symptomatic treatment is the rule. Children should be kept in bed until the temperature returns to normal. They should be given plenty of liquids to drink. Light snacks may be offered when the child gets hungry. If the doctor approves, some medication may be given to reduce fever and relieve the pain of headaches. Aspirin should be avoided because of its apparent connection to REYE'S SYNDROME when a child has the flu.

Inner Ear Infection

See EAR INFECTIONS

Intestinal Obstruction

An interference with the normal flow of contents through the intestinal tract.

Obstructions may be partial or complete, mechanical or metabolic. Strangulated HERNIAS, bands or adhesions, INTUSSUSCEPTION, and congenital (present-at-birth) abnormalities of intestinal formation are the most common causes in infancy and childhood. Occasionally a new-born baby's bowels will be plugged by too much meconium (a substance created in the intestinal tract while the baby is in the uterus). In rare cases, tumors or parasites may be involved, and at times certain infections such as PNEUMONIA or PERITONITIS may cause an intestinal obstruction.

An infant or child whose intestine is blocked looks very ill. Cramping abdominal pain develops early. Vomiting is usually present and abdominal bloating, a later sign, may be severe. Fevers, respiration that alternates between slow and rapid, and extreme paleness indicate the seriousness of the problem.

ACTION — If the block is mechanical, it must be relieved, often by surgery. Metabolic or infectious causes must also be medically treated in a vigorous fashion to avoid complications that are a direct threat to life.

See also PYLORIC STENOSIS

Intussusception

A form of intestinal obstruction in which one portion of the intestine "telescopes" over another.

Although no age group is immune to intussusception, the condition generally occurs in infants and children under the age of two. It is somewhat more common in boys than in girls.

A child suffers from periods of intense cramping and often screams in pain. The cramping is cyclic in nature, with a period of relief for 15 or 20 minutes and then a crying out. Sometimes a large, jellylike, bloody bowel movement is passed.

ACTION — Intussusception is a medical emergency because the blockage impedes blood flow, allowing gangrene to set in. It must be corrected before that happens. Surgery is the most common approach, but a nonsurgical technique involving the rectal introduction of barium may be effective when it alters hydrostatic pressure at the site of intussusception.

J

Jock Itch

The common name for a fungus infection that causes a scaling, itchy rash in the groin area.

Jock itch is rare in children and uncommon in females. However, it can occur in young people, especially adolescent boys. Hot, humid climates and tight-fitting clothing seem to contribute to growth of the fungus, which causes a bright red rash with a very sharp border.

ACTION — The application of special antifungal solutions or creams helps, as does wearing loose-fitting clothes.

Juvenile Rheumatoid Arthritis

Also known as Still's disease, this condition is similar to rheumatoid arthritis in adults.

Typical signs and symptoms of juvenile rheumatoid arthritis include painful and swollen joints (especially larger joints), skin rashes, and swollen lymph glands. A physician may note an enlarged liver and spleen.

Children are often sickest during the development stage of juvenile rheumatoid arthritis. The body temperature may rise to about 105° F (40° C) and stay that high for several weeks. In some cases, there is an associated inflammation of the lungs and the membranes that cover the heart. The child will be lethargic and complain of malaise (a generalized feeling of being unwell). In some cases, there may be an interference with normal growth and development; this sometimes involves the lower jaw, creating a receding chin line.

Juvenile rheumatoid arthritis may occur in early childhood, but rarely before the age of 2 years. In school-age children, it may develop between the ages of 8 and 12. It is more common in girls than in boys.

ACTION — Although the outlook is good compared with that for adult rheumatoid arthritis, it is a serious and chronic disease that may require physical therapy to help maintain joint mobility and good muscle tone, as well as, in many cases, supportive counseling to help the child and the parents cope with the nature of the disease and the probable need for long-term therapy.

Treatment is aimed at relieving symptoms and preventing deterioration of the joints. If the latter can be achieved, normal adulthood can be anticipated, since the disease tends to disappear when the child matures. Aspirin or acetaminophen is generally recommended for the relief of symptoms. Occasionally short courses of steroid therapy may be used.

Physical therapy is aimed at preventing permanent deformity or the wasting of muscles. The child and the parents will most likely be taught certain exercises that can be performed at home.

As to emotional impact, the child's doctor or a recommended psychotherapist may be helpful in teaching both the child and the parents how to live with juvenile rheumatoid arthritis.

K

Kidney Infections and Diseases

A BACTERIAL INFECTION *affecting a child's kidney tissue or the collecting system that transfers urine to the bladder.*

Unlike CYSTITIS, kidney infections are frequently associated with high fever and back pain. The child may look quite ill. Abdominal pain and vomiting often make an appearance. The child goes to the bathroom frequently, experiences a burning sensation on urinating, and the urine voided may appear cloudy or bloody.

Nephritis, the technical term for a kidney inflammation, is not always a result of infection. Sometimes the inflammation seems to start without a known cause, becoming constant and gradually progressing to kidney failure. Some cases are acute and do not become chronic. Some cases are associated with other diseases or seem to have a hereditary basis or, as in acute glomerulonephritis, may occur because of a previous strep infection.

A disease called *nephrosis* sometimes occurs in preschool children; it is somewhat more common in boys than in girls. No one is sure what causes it, but it usually starts with a gradual weight gain that reflects edema, the slow but sure accumulation of fluids in the tissues of the body. Although puffiness around the eyes is fairly common early in the disease, the weight gain is often first thought to be normal growth.

ACTION — For infections: To avoid long-term kidney damage, a doctor must be consulted. The doctor takes the child's medical history and does a physical examination and lab tests, because diagnosis requires findings such as pus in the urine and the growth of bacteria in a culture specimen. Once the acute condition is under control, x-rays may be taken and the inside of the bladder may be checked by cystoscopic examination to make sure there is no obstruction to urinary flow, which could cause a backup of pressure against kidney tissue.

For nephritis: Once chronic nephritis has severely damaged the kidney, there is nothing that can be done to repair the problem. The child may have to be connected to a dialysis machine several times a week. This machine has tubes that connect with the patient's blood system, so that waste products can be filtered out before the now-purified blood is recirculated.

An alternative method involves surgical transplantation of a normal kidney. This technique requires careful matching and the use of potent medications to minimize the chance of rejection. The operation is effective, sometimes permitting normal functioning over a period of many years. However, side effects can occur, and for many people the cost remains prohibitive.

For nephrosis: Antibiotic and corticosteroid or immunosuppressive drugs are generally prescribed, as well as diuretics (medications that make one urinate more frequently) to keep down the excess fluid. Nutritional guidance is usually necessary, as children with nephrosis often lose their appetites. It is especially important for the child to maintain a diet that is low in salt. Also, because infections can cause relapses, parents are generally advised to let the doctor know immediately if the child shows any signs of infection, such as a cough or fever. Finally, some family counseling may be helpful, because children with nephrosis must take special care not to expose themselves to infection, yet they should not be allowed to become loners and should be encouraged to lead as normal a life as possible.

More information is available by calling the American Kidney Fund at 800-638-8299 (800-492-8361 in Maryland).

Kissing Disease

See INFECTIOUS MONONUCLEOSIS

Knock-Knees

A posture of the legs in which the knees come together and the lower legs flare outward.

During growth at the toddler stage, it is normal for the knees at times to seem too close together. Even if the deformity is marked, it generally corrects itself as the child gets older. On rare occasion rickets or a congenital (present-at-birth) bone disorder may cause abnormalities of the knee joint.

ACTION — Only if ligaments around the knee are being stretched is any aggressive therapy, such as bracing, recommended. Even then the knees do not straighten; all that happens is that further relaxation of the ligaments is prevented. Wedges in shoes do not correct the defect.

Compare BOWLEGS

L

Laryngitis

Inflammation of the larynx (the voice box).

An acute attack of laryngitis can develop suddenly because of overusing the voice, as in shouting, cheering, singing, or otherwise abusing the vocal cords. Laryngitis may also develop from an upper-respiratory VIRAL INFECTION such as the COMMON COLD, BRONCHITIS, TONSILLITIS, sore throat, SINUSITIS, PERTUSSIS (whooping cough), or MEASLES.

Symptoms include hoarseness, a tickling sensation or pain in the throat, difficulty in swallowing, and, if the larynx is swollen, short-ness of breath on physical exertion or other breathing difficulties.

Chronic laryngitis can result from inadequate treatment of repeat acute attacks or from starting to overuse the voice again before the larynx has fully healed. Swollen tissues may become thickened with scar tissue, leading to permanent damage to the voice. Irritants, including smoke, can lead to further thickening of the vocal cords and cartilage tissues of the larynx.

ACTION — Laryngitis will usually clear up with voice rest and steam inhalation. Laryngitis can be an early sign of CROUP. If severe, croup demands a doctor's careful examination and treatment. Sometimes antibiotics are prescribed to treat any associated bacterial infection.

Lazy Eye

See STRABISMUS

Leukemia

A form of cancer in which there is an abnormal, uncontrolled multi-plication of leukocytes (immature white blood cells).

These cells cannot function normally, and they also eventually infil-trate other tissues, such as bone marrow, preventing the production of the other components of normal blood. The failure of red cell formation leads to ANEMIA, the immaturity of the white cells lowers the body's resistance to infection, and the lack of platelet production increases the risk of abnormal bleeding. Therefore anemia, infection, and bleed-ing are common signs.

Fairly early on the child with acute lymphatic leukemia shows increased fatigue, a pale complexion, unexplained fever, repeated in-fections, and an abnormal amount of bruising that cannot be ac-counted for. The examining physician will probably note an enlarged liver or spleen. Laboratory findings generally include a large increase in white blood cells, many of which are immature, and lowered red cell and platelet counts. The confirming diagnosis is made by examining a specimen of bone marrow.

The acute lymphatic type of leukemia accounts for about 80 per-cent of all childhood cases. There are several forms of the disease, such as acute lymphocytic leukemia (ALL), acute granulocytic leuke-mia (AGL), and acute meyloid leukemia (AML), which is much more common in adults.

ACTION — Current treatment, such as chemotherapy, transfusions, and antibiotics to fight associated bacterial infections, allows about 90 percent of the children to enjoy a period of remission, in which symptoms temporarily go away, and now many survive longer than five years after diagnosis. Since leukemia is potentially a fatal disease, the parents, the child, and any siblings may benefit greatly from counseling that helps them understand the disease's impact and how they can participate most actively in the course of treatment.

Lockjaw

See TETANUS

Low Blood Sugar

See HYPOGLYCEMIA

Lupus Erythematosus

A chronic disease of unknown origin that is both systemic (affecting large portions of the body) and cutaneous (affecting the skin). It is considered a collagen disease (collagen is the supportive material that holds skin, tendons, bones, cartilage, and connective tissue together).

Lupus erythematosus is thought to be an autoimmune disease, that is, one in which the body's natural defense system malfunctions and produces antibodies against some of the sufferer's own tissue.

The disease is not common in children, but when it does occur it is usually more acute and more serious than in adults. Early symptoms include fever, pain and inflammation of the joints, and skin rash. In some cases, a red patch forms on the face and over the bridge of the nose (the so-called butterfly rash). The skin eruptions may spread to the neck, chest, and extremities, although only about one third of the children with lupus experience this effect, which is worsened by exposure to sunlight. Many children experience malaise (a general feeling of being unwell), loss of appetite, and loss of weight.

Systemic lupus erythematosus, also known as disseminated lupus, is a progressive and potentially fatal disease that can affect the functioning of the lungs, kidneys, and heart. Treatment depends on the severity of the disease and which organs are affected. A particularly dangerous complication in children is the development of nephritis (inflammation of the kidneys).

ACTION — For systemic lupus erythematosus, corticosteroids are generally prescribed. Modern treatment methods allow more than 85 percent of lupus-stricken children to survive for at least 10 years, and some may escape the fatal outcome that was once prevalent.

Milder forms of the disease have an even more favorable outlook. Topical steroid preparations can be used for facial rash, and other drugs are prescribed to relieve pain and inflammation of affected joints. Antimalarial drugs such as hydroxychloroquine are sometimes useful. The main goal is to relieve symptoms and to control or suppress any associated disease of the kidneys or other internal organs.

Lyme Disease

A bacterial infection transmitted by the deer tick; in the United States, it is found predominantly in the Northern and Northeastern regions.

Although this disease — which has been around for years but was first noted as a distinct illness in Lyme, Connecticut, in 1975 — has become a hot item on newscasts and in the press and a great worry to parents, it is relatively rare.

In nature, certain animals, including deer and mice, may be infected with the disease that causes Lyme in children and adults. Ticks suck the blood of these animals and, when humans wander into rural areas covered with high grasses and bushes, the ticks that live there latch onto unprotected skin and, while sucking the human blood, pass on the parasite from the diseased animals.

Although Lyme disease manifests itself in a number of ways — often leading to misdiagnosis (frequently as INFECTIOUS MONONUCLEOSIS) and overdiagnosis — a vast majority of the time the first sign is a rash forming a ring around the tick bite, accompanied by INFLUENZA-like symptoms such as high fever, headache, general fatigue and achiness, and loss of appetite. In later stages, more serious complications may arise involving the heart, the brain (MENINGITIS), and the joints (producing an ARTHRITIS-like pain).

ACTION — A child showing Lyme symptoms should be taken as soon as possible to a doctor, who will draw blood for tests to confirm the diagnosis. Treatment, begun in the disease's early stages, should cure it. Some cases, however, may resist the treatments, or the blood test may not pick up the disease in its early stages; therefore, some cases may reach the later stages with more serious complications.

Antibiotics such as tetracycline and penicillin prescribed by the child's physician or health-care professional usually take care of the problem. If the disease is in its later stages, higher dosages or stronger medications may be necessary.

Prevention is the safest course. When children go into wooded and grassy areas, be sure they wear clothing that will protect them from errant ticks. Even if the weather is warm, long-sleeved shirts, long pants, high socks, and other clothes that cover most of the skin are recommended. Not recommended, however, are insect repellents containing DEET; children exposed repeatedly to such chemicals may experience a wide array of potential side effects from skin rashes to neurological damage.

Lymphangitis

Inflammation of lymphatic channels or vessels.

As the lymphatic system tries to remove or drain off infection, lymph channels may become inflamed, creating thick red lines. Occasionally the lymph glands that drain an area of infection become swollen and tender.

ACTION — In rare instances, the original site of infection may need to be drained surgically. Usually antibiotics cure the infection, and the red streaks disappear.

See also SWOLLEN GLANDS

M

Malabsorption Syndrome

Any of a variety of conditions that affect the intestines or digestive glands in such a way that causes some failure in absorption of one or more nutrients essential for health.

The most common sign, called *steatorrhea*, is the passing of loose stools that contain excessive fat. The stools are pale, bulky, and so light that they may require several flushes for complete toilet disposal. Other signs and symptoms include weight loss, abdominal bloating, muscle wasting, anorexia (diminished appetite), and audible gurgling or splashing sounds coming from the intestine.

A specific, although fairly uncommon, example of a malabsorption disorder is called *celiac disease* or *nontropical sprue*. It tends to run in families, and children as young as six months old may be affected. If it is left untreated, celiac disease of childhood is typified by abdominal bloating, steatorrhea, muscle wasting, loss of appetite, severe diarrhea, stunted growth, and general listlessness. In celiac disease, the digestive tract cannot tolerate gluten, a component of wheat and other cereals. In some way not yet understood, gluten damages the lining of the intestines in those who are sensitive to the substance.

ACTION — Because malabsorption syndromes occur with different frequencies at different ages (some may be discovered shortly after birth), and because treatment is based on the specific underlying cause, parents are urged to seek medical evaluation of any child who seems to be showing signs of malnourishment and/or marked gastrointestinal upset. The treatment of celiac disease is simple: Avoid gluten; the results are dramatically good. However, avoiding gluten may not be easy because, in addition to the more obvious foods such as wheat flour and cereals, it may be present in cakes, cookies, and bread. The child's doctor can provide parents with a list of foods and recipes that are gluten free.

Malignancy

See CANCER

Mastitis

See BREASTS, DISEASES/CONDITIONS OF

Mastoiditis

Inflammation of any part of the mastoid process — that prominent piece of spongy bone just behind the earlobe.

The mastoid's air cavities lead directly to the middle ear, so middle ear infections sometimes spread to the mastoid process.

An early symptom of mastoiditis is intense pain behind the ear. The child's temperature may rise slightly, the pulse rate may become rapid, there may be a discharge from the affected ear, and hearing loss will be fairly pronounced. If an abscess develops within the mastoid's air cells, swelling behind the ear can be quite noticeable.

ACTION — Before the days of antibiotic therapy, mastoiditis often meant surgical removal of a section of bone so that pus could be drained. Today the early diagnosis and treatment of EAR INFECTIONS means that the mastoid process is less frequently affected. Even when it is, antibiotic therapy, generally continued over a period of two weeks, is quite effective. Only in advanced cases in which the child has not received appropriate medical treatment might there be a need for surgical drainage.

As with any ear problem, the child should be taken to a doctor as soon as the slightest indication of mastoiditis appears. This reduces the risk of further complications, including possibly MENINGITIS.

MBD

See ATTENTION-DEFICIT DISORDERS

Measles

A highly contagious VIRAL INFECTION *with a typical red skin rash and grain-sized white spots on a red base on the mouth (called Koplik's spots).*

The incubation period for measles is about 10 to 14 days. First signs are fever, runny nose, red and watery eyes, sneezing, and a hacking cough. The temperature generally continues to rise slightly every day for about three or four days and may go as high as 104° F (40° C). It is about this time that the typical oral rash (Koplik's spots) may sometimes be seen on the inner surface of the cheeks; the spots appear and disappear rapidly, usually within 12 to 18 hours.

The skin rash begins behind the ears and spreads to the face and neck. Within the next day or two, it spreads to the body and limbs, becomes blotchy in places, increases in size, and changes to a slightly darker color.

The eyes of children with measles are especially sensitive to light for the first few days. It is not necessary to darken the room, but strong lights should be avoided.

Most cases of measles present no serious problems, but the doctor will want to make sure that there is not also an infection of the eyes, ears, or lungs. In very rare instances, bleeding from the mouth, nose, or bowels (hemorrhagic measles) may develop. Parents should immediately call the child's doctor if this happens.

Be sure your child is vaccinated against measles. Despite the availability of measles vaccines, many parents are not making sure their children are getting those immunization shots or getting them at the proper times. Because of this, the incidence of measles cases increased more than 73 percent from 1989 to 1990, and nearly half of those cases involved children under the age of five.

ACTION — Aside from relieving symptoms, there is little treatment for measles — other than prevention by prior immunization. Because it is caused by a virus, it does not respond to antibiotics. A recent study suggested that giving a measles-infected child vitamin A may speed recovery and reduce risks of fatality because measles tends to deplete vitamin A in the body.

If the child's eyelids tend to stick together, the doctor may prescribe some special eyedrops. When the fever is high, cool sponging offers some relief, and the child should be offered tempting liquids frequently.

See IMMUNIZATION

Compare RUBELLA, CHICKEN POX

Meckel's Diverticulum

A small outpouching of the intestinal wall, at the far end of the small intestine. The defect occurs when a duct normally present before birth fails to disappear altogether.

A Meckel's diverticulum may cause problems if the tissue becomes irritated and bleeds or perforates. Its presence is often determined only after a search for the cause of ANEMIA is made.

Bleeding may be slow and scant in amount, and rarely is it associated with pain. When it does occur, abdominal pain is vague and centers around the navel. On some occasions a Meckel's diverticulum may cause an INTESTINAL OBSTRUCTION, and if the inflammation is severe or a perforation is present, the child may show symptoms resembling those of acute APPENDICITIS.

ACTION — The only cure for Meckel's diverticulum is surgery.

Meningitis

Inflammation of the meninges, the three delicate membranes that cover the brain.

Meningitis is generally caused by bacterial or viral microorganisms, the latter called aseptic meningitis. These infections often spread to the meninges from other sites such as the ears, sinuses, tonsils, or upper-respiratory tract. The first symptoms are common to many other infections: high temperature, chills, severe headache, and vomiting. Lethargy and irritability are common. Marked stiffness of the neck is a prominent sign; the child's head may bend back and he or she may not be able to bend it forward. Infants may show a bulging fontanel or soft spot, and as pressure within the skull increases, they may cry out in a shrill, high-pitched tone. Convulsions may occur, as well as coma. Children with meningitis may also be in a state of blood-system shock if the bacteria get into the bloodstream. A purplish rash, caused by widespread blockage of small blood vessels, may occur.

ACTION — Immediate medical attention is required for this serious condition. Hospitalization is the rule, and the medical team will most likely do a spinal tap, that is, take a sample of cerebrospinal fluid (fluid in the spinal canal) to confirm the diagnosis. It will be analyzed not only for specific organisms but also for the prevalence of certain white blood cells, protein content, sugar content, and other diagnostic signs.

Antibiotic treatment is used. With prompt and proper treatment, the chances of complete and uncomplicated recovery from meningitis are very good.

In late 1990, the U.S. Department of Health and Human Services urged physicians to give infants as young as two months of age anti-Hemophilus influenza type B vaccinations along with their DTP and polio immunizations in order to guard against Hemophilus-caused meningitis. Such meningitis attacks more than 5,000 infants per year; 800 die from it, while nearly 40 percent of the survivors show neurological complications such as blindness, deafness, paralysis, and retardation.

Compare ENCEPHALITIS

Milk Allergy

An allergic reaction to one or more of the proteins in cow's milk. The disorder is sometimes called "cow's milk protein sensitivity."

In infants from birth to about six months, typical signs and symptoms are fever, vomiting, diarrhea (with watery stools sometimes tinged with blood), steatorrhea (excessive amounts of fat in bowel movements), weight loss or failure to gain weight, and ANEMIA. Some babies may develop severe and persistent diarrhea that directly interferes with the absorption of essential nutrients by the small intestines. In rare cases, the infant may even experience ANAPHYLACTIC SHOCK.

A second basic form of milk allergy is usually first noted when the hypersensitive child is between the ages of six months and two years. Signs and symptoms may include wheezing, nasal congestion, swelling, constant or intermittent diarrhea, and a failure to thrive resulting from the digestive tract's failure to absorb nutrient proteins properly.

ACTION — Once the diagnosis is made, cow's milk must be eliminated from the child's diet for a period of time. It can be replaced with a special hypoallergenic formula. If the symptoms disappear and the child once again reacts badly to cow's milk, the diagnosis is confirmed and the youngster is placed back on the hypoallergenic formula. It is advised that any milk challenges be done very cautiously, and only under the guidance of a physician.

For reasons not clearly understood, many of these children are able to tolerate cow's milk once they grow older. Most pediatricians recommend that children be kept on the hypoallergenic formula for at least one year before cow's milk is reintroduced into their diets.

See also ALLERGY, LACTASE DEFICIENCY, LACTOSE INTOLERANCE

Minimal Brain Dysfunction

See ATTENTION-DEFICIT DISORDERS

Mongolism

See DOWN'S SYNDROME

Moniliasis

See THRUSH, YEAST INFECTION

Mononucleosis

See INFECTIOUS MONONUCLEOSIS

Motion Sickness

Sometimes called "travel sickness," this is sensitivity of the equilibrium center, which, when activated, can lead to nausea, dizziness, and even vomiting, and can take several hours to pass.

Motion sickness is caused by the effects of irregular or rhythmic movements as they cause two small motion detectors in the inner ear to do "flip-flops."

Action — Ways to try to prevent a child falling prey to motion sickness during a long car trip include having the child sit in the front seat instead of the back and having the child keep looking through the windshield instead of looking down to read books or play games.

Often children outgrow the tendency toward motion sickness. Until they do, parents can ensure more comfortable trips by administering children's doses of nonprescription antihistamine products such as Antivert, Bonine, Dramamine, Emetrol, Marezine, Tigan, Trave-Arex, or Vertrol about an hour before traveling; these drugs may last for up to six hours. As with any medication, it is essential that label instructions be followed to the letter and that very young children not be given some medications. When in doubt, call the child's doctor or health-care professional for advice.

If sickness does occur, parents should not chastise, punish, or tease a child who becomes motion sick. There is nothing the child can do to stop the situation.

Mumps

A VIRAL INFECTION *of the salivary glands located along the jaw that especially affects the parotid gland, located just in front of the ear.*

The virus can be spread through the breath of an infected child, who may then transmit the disease within 48 hours even though he or she will not come down with the disease until the incubation period of two or three weeks has passed. Because of its long incubation period, mumps spreads throughout a family or a school long before individual sufferers show signs of the disease.

Children between the ages of 5 and 15 are most susceptible, although it is possible to catch mumps at any age. One bout of mumps normally provides protection for life; there is also an immunization shot that should be given to anyone over the age of 15 months.

First signs of mumps are stiffness and slight pain in the neck, followed by a swelling of the parotid gland, which greatly enlarges the entire side of the neck and cheek, usually on one side but sometimes on both. A child may have difficulty opening the mouth, the mouth may become quite dry, and fever is present. In severe cases, there may be vomiting, and the temperature can go as high as 104° F (40° C).

Most cases of mumps are relatively mild, discounting the neck discomfort, and the swelling usually recedes in five to ten days. Complications are rare in young children, but adolescents may sometimes get an infection of the pancreas, thyroid gland, testicles, or ovaries. When complications do occur in childhood, they may be in the form of ENCEPHALITIS (an inflammation of the brain). However, this occurs in only about 250 out of 100,000 cases and carries a mortality rate of only about 2 percent in those who contract encephalitis.

ACTION — There is no special therapy other than keeping the mouth clean and refreshed with gargles or mouthwashes and offering plenty of liquids. Some children get some relief of discomfort if a hot-water bottle is placed along the neck; others prefer an ice pack. Parents can apply whichever feels better to the child.

Murmurs

See HEART MURMURS

Muscular Dystrophy

A group of disorders characterized by gradual and progressive degeneration (wasting away) of muscle fibers, which eventually causes crippling.

The exact origin of muscular dystrophy is not clear, but at least half of those children suffering from the disease have a family history in which at least one member of the direct family line, of either sex, is affected. It is thought to be associated with an inherited difficulty in the ability of muscles to take up amino acid (a protein) and use it as a source of repair and growth energy. This probably occurs because of an enzyme deficiency. The result is atrophy (muscle wasting) instead of growth. Classification depends on age of onset, the rate at which weakness progresses, and how the muscular involvement is distributed throughout the body.

Boys are affected more often than girls. Sometimes the youngster waddles like a duck, has trouble climbing stairs, and falls frequently. The muscles of the chest, abdomen, and buttocks are affected first; then the disease progresses steadily to involve other body parts. As a general rule, disability is fastest in children in whom the disease appears early in life — at or before the age of 3. Most children with muscular dystrophy are confined to a wheelchair by the time they are 10 or 12.

ACTION — There is no cure and no specific treatment for this group of diseases. Strenuous exercise should be avoided because it can hasten the breakdown of muscle fibers. On the other hand, children should be kept moderately active and walking for as long as possible, both for psychological reasons and to minimize muscle contractures and deformities. To keep the child functioning fairly normally for as long as possible, it is necessary to enlist the aid of many people, including school personnel, who may be able to help arrange for transportation and see to special needs, such as toilet facilities for the child. Diet should be low in calories to help prevent too much weight gain. All infections, especially upper-respiratory infections, should be treated promptly, since the child with muscular dystrophy develops difficulty in expanding the chest and/or coughing. Counseling with experts in the field may be useful to the entire family, for muscular dystrophy afflicts not only the affected child but everyone who is close to the child.

Myopia

See NEARSIGHTEDNESS

N

Nearsightedness

A visual disorder called myopia, which occurs when the eyeball is too long from front to back.

When light enters the eye, it falls short and is focused at a point in front of the retina. This causes a blurred image because the light rays disperse again before they actually reach the retina. Objects nearby can be seen far more clearly, which accounts for the name nearsightedness.

Unlike FARSIGHTEDNESS, nearsightedness is rarely present at birth. It usually becomes evident in school-age children, who are seen holding books or other objects close to their eyes in order to achieve proper focusing. The prevalence of myopia increases during childhood, peaking somewhere between the ages of 8 and 14.

ACTION — It is important for school-age children to have at least annual eye exams. If a school's screening program reveals any problem, the child should immediately be taken to an eye specialist so that appropriate corrective lenses can be prescribed.

Nephritis

See KIDNEY INFECTIONS AND DISEASES

Nephrosis

See KIDNEY INFECTIONS AND DISEASES

O

Otitis

See EAR INFECTIONS

Outer Ear Infection

See EAR INFECTIONS

P

Panic Attack

A sudden overwhelming feeling of extreme and irrational anxiety.

In a general way, anxiety may be differentiated from fear. The latter is usually aroused by some readily observable object, event, or set of circumstances that the child can understandably or justifiably perceive as frightening. Anxiety may occur in response to seemingly trivial things: a noise on the radio, a buzzing fly, a blinking light; or as a result of some inner experience of a physiological or psychological nature.

Because the autonomic nervous system — the one that controls involuntary processes such as breathing — discharges or fires impulses so rapidly, the child may perspire, look pale, shake, and show rapid breathing and a fast heart rate.

Children stricken by this panic may feel dizzy, faint, or numb; fear dying; or experience choking or smothering sensations. Occasionally, they may fear that they are going crazy.

ACTION — Calm reassurance may be of some help, but repeated episodes should warn the parent that a medical evaluation is needed. It has recently been found that these panic attacks may be associated with metabolic disease, and medication may be helpful.

Peritonitis

Inflammation of the peritoneum.

The peritoneum is the thin, smooth, almost transparent, moist membrane that lines the walls of the abdominal cavity and parts of internal organs. The peritoneum provides a smooth surface upon which organs can glide as they undergo natural movement and slight changes of shape.

117

Before the advent of antibiotics, peritonitis was severely life threatening. Even now, it remains an extremely serious condition that requires immediate medical attention.

In children, the most common cause is a ruptured appendix. However, any condition that allows a spread of bacterial infection in the abdominal cavity can cause peritonitis. For example, a penetrating wound or a perforated large intestine may release bacteria-containing waste matter that can infect the entire peritoneal area. The inflammation can also be caused by the abnormal release of irritating body substances, such as bile, urine, blood, or digestive juices, into the abdominal cavity. Because female internal reproductive organs are so closely associated with the peritoneum, infection there can also spread.

The child with peritonitis may experience nausea and vomiting, fever, chills, abdominal bloating, and diffuse abdominal pain so severe that the slightest movement may worsen the pain. Muscular contractions that normally move intestinal contents may stop, so the child suffers constipation and a painful rigidity of abdominal muscles.

ACTION — Once the parent has the slightest suspicion of peritonitis, absolutely no food and no laxatives should be given. The child's doctor or a medical emergency facility should be consulted immediately.

The child should be hospitalized so that antibiotics can be injected and nutrient fluids can be fed intravenously until healing occurs. If rupture or perforation of the intestinal tract or another body organ occurs, surgery is necessary to repair the affected organ.

Pertussis

A highly contagious BACTERIAL INFECTION, *commonly called whooping cough.*

Pertussis is spread in the air from the breath or cough of an infected person and causes complications such as PNEUMONIA, inflamed intestines, and convulsions. It is most serious in babies under one year of age.

The first signs of whooping cough begin about one or two weeks after exposure to the germs. For several days or a week it seems to be just a bad chest cold with coughing. During the second week, the coughing increases, coming in series of spasms between cough-free intervals. Children may cough several times very rapidly, "whooping" in an effort to catch their breath. The high-pitched, rasping sound is caused by air being sucked in over the vocal cords, which are covered with mucus. Spitting out some of the mucus relieves the attack for a time. Young infants are generally unable to clear this mucus. In fact, they may not show typical symptoms, such as whooping, but they are apt to suffer sudden bouts of extreme difficulty in breathing, whereupon they turn a bluish color.

Coughing and whooping may last for six weeks or more, but generally the intensity and frequency taper after about the fourth week.

Despite the wide availability of an affordable pertussis immunization vaccine, a study by the Centers for Disease Control (CDC) found that of children between the ages of three months and four years who contracted pertussis, 63 percent had not been properly immunized, and 34 percent had never received the vaccine at all.

ACTION — The child's doctor should be consulted promptly during the early stages of the illness. At times, suctioning of mucus and oxygen therapy are required. In severe cases, antibiotics may be prescribed, although they do not shorten the time a child has the disease. For the most part, tender loving care is the best treatment. The child should be kept in bed while symptoms are severe; later he or she can be up and about, although isolated from other children to whom the disease might spread. Feedings should be limited to frequent small helpings rather than large meals, and plenty of liquids should be offered, since they may help somewhat to thin the mucous secretions. In young children, solid foods should be restricted until the violent coughing begins to subside.

Children can be, and should be, protected from whooping cough by the DPT vaccination, one of the routine immunizations of childhood. However, there are certain children at high risk of having an IMMUNIZATION REACTION to the pertussis portion of the DPT shot who should avoid it. According to the CDC, those at highest risk are those children:

• Who are over seven years old
• Who have a fever-related illness
• With a history of convulsions
• Undergoing immunosuppressive therapy
• With a neurological disorder

Even the above may not be absolute contraindications, and immunization may be given on the recommendation of the child's physician.

See IMMUNIZATION

Phenylketonuria

An inherited (genetically determined) disorder, often referred to by the initials PKU, in which a child is deficient in an enzyme that helps the body process an essential amino acid called phenylalanine.

Fortunately, screening for PKU in newborn babies is now an extremely widespread practice in developed countries; most states within the United States require it by law. Two popular PKU screening tests are the Guthrie bacterial inhibition test and the chromatography technique. Both start with a tiny sample of the infant's blood, usually obtained by pricking the heel. If the laboratory analysis shows an elevated amount of phenylalanine, more sophisticated diagnostic tests are done to confirm the diagnosis.

When phenylketonuria is not detected and treated early, children are brain damaged by the excess chemical they cannot process. Symptoms of undetected PKU include mental retardation, seizures, and ECZEMA (a generalized rash). Affected children usually have fair hair and skins (because phenylalanine inhibits the production of pigment); poor eating habits, with failure to thrive; and urine that has a peculiar odor.

PKU is a comparatively rare condition, occurring in about 1 in 10,000 births, but because it is a genetic defect, parents of a PKU infant may wish to seek genetic counseling about future plans for more children. PKU is carried by a recessive, not a dominant, gene. If two people both carrying the recessive gene choose to have a family, statistically one fourth of their children will have PKU; one fourth will be entirely free of both the disease and the genetic trait; but one half will themselves be carriers of the recessive trait for PKU, which means they could pass the disease or the trait to the following generation.

ACTION — The child with phenylketonuria is placed on a special diet that provides little phenylalanine. Part of the diet is a milk substitute, such as LoFenolac. Fruits, vegetables, and other foods low in phenylalanine are also recommended. Many authorities now contend that this special diet can be altered or even discontinued altogether about the time the child is ready for school, which is convenient timing, since as children become older, it is more difficult for parents to successfully restrict their diets.

Pigeon Chest

A deformity in which an overgrowth of breastbone-to-ribs cartilage causes an outward displacement of the chest.

In some infants the condition may be associated with congenital (present-at-birth) heart disease. Up to about age six, it may be associated with ASTHMA. However, as a general rule, there is no interference with heart or lung functions, and there seems to be no definite cause of pigeon chest. Most cases appear in adolescence, when, with seeming suddenness, the chest wall may jut out six inches or so.

ACTION — If the deformity is severe, it will have very definite psychological implications. Cosmetic surgery can permanently restore normal chest contour, so if the child is of an appropriate age (as determined by a qualified surgeon), parents should give careful consideration to enhancing their child's chances for a life no longer marred by physical disability.

Compare SUNKEN CHEST

Pinkeye

See CONJUNCTIVITIS

Pinworms

Also known as threadworms, pinworms are the most common worm infestation that children experience.

Especially in warm climates, pinworm infestation is an extremely common childhood ailment and one parents should not feel embarrassed about; it does not suggest a lack of household or personal cleanliness.

At one time or another, at least 20 percent of all children are infested with pinworms, which are harbored in the cecum, an intestinal pouch from which the appendix arises. The female worm travels down to the large intestine and rectum to lay her tiny eggs on the region around the anus. Eggs are passed from children's fingers into children's mouths (their own or those of playmates). The swallowed eggs go back down into the intestine, where they are hatched, and then the whole cycle is repeated.

Some children have no symptoms and signs, although occasionally abdominal pain, possibly mistaken for APPENDICITIS, may occur. Many children recover spontaneously, provided reinfestation does not occur.

If children do have symptoms, they most likely complain of anal itching. This can become quite intense, and the whole area may become painful and reddened if the child scratches. Sleep may be restless and uncomfortable, especially shortly after the child goes to bed.

ACTION — There are two methods to discover worms or eggs. After the child has been in bed asleep for a couple of hours, use a flashlight to examine the anal area. Pinworms are threadlike little creatures, quite small but visible to the naked eye. Another method, performed by a physician, involves using tape to pat the child's anal region. The strip of transparent tape, attached facedown to a glass slide, can then be examined in a lab or a doctor's office to see if eggs are present.

Pyrantel pamoate, peperazine citrate, mebendazole, and other anthelmintics (intestinal worm killers) are generally prescribed, and the doctor may choose to treat the entire family because the infection is so highly contagious. Although some doctors suggest extra hygienic precautions, many authorities believe that meticulous standards of cleanliness, such as repeated hand washing, have little effect on the control or prevention of pinworm infestation.

PKU

See PHENYLKETONURIA

Pleurisy

Inflammation of the pleura (the membrane that covers the outside of the lungs and the inner side of the ribs).

Pleurisy is not particularly common these days, probably because it generally appears as a complication of some other condition such as rib injury or PNEUMONIA, which nowadays is usually effectively treated before pleurisy sets in.

The disorder called dry pleurisy begins suddenly with very severe pain in the side, which becomes even worse when the child takes deep breaths, coughs, or moves. The pain is caused because the surfaces of the pleural membrane move against each other. A slight fever may be present. If the inflammation is mild, the pain will disappear in two or three days and the child will recover rapidly.

If considerable fluid builds up — a condition called pleurisy with effusion — there will be less pain because the walls of the pleural membrane separate, but shortness of breath may occur. If the situation is left unattended, the excess fluid may cause collapse of a lung. The fluid may also begin to exude pus in a condition called purulent pleurisy, which can cause the child to cough up pus-tinged mucus.

ACTION — When parents suspect pleurisy, they should check with the child's doctor. In extreme cases, it may be necessary to drain accumulated fluid.

Pneumonia

An inflammation of the lungs, typically accompanied by a collection of fluid in the alveoli (air sacs) of the affected tissue.

Pneumonia can range from a small patch in one lung to extensive involvement of both lungs, called *double pneumonia*. Very mild and limited cases often go undetected, and the child recovers completely.

Doctors classify pneumonia two ways: by the nature of the infection, usually viral or bacterial, and by the extent of the infection. *Lobar pneumonia* simply means that a major division of a lung, called a lobe, is involved. Bronchopneumonia has spread from a bronchus (one of the lung's major air passages), and an x-ray will show a series of small solid patches of affected lung tissue rather than one large, dense area, as in lobar pneumonia. INFLUENZA, acute BRONCHITIS, PERTUSSIS, and MEASLES are among the common predecessors.

Although less common than viruses or bacteria, other causes include fungi; the accidental inhalation of food particles, vomitus, or pus from an upper-respiratory infection; or inhaling irritating gases or chemicals. Newborn babies occasionally contract pneumonia from aspirating meconium (a substance created in the intestinal tract while the baby is in the uterus). Babies born in a modern hospital have the advantage of immediate medical attention for this problem, and the condition usually clears up without complications.

Pneumonia used to be extremely dangerous in young children.

Currently, with prompt diagnosis and treatment, the child often recovers in less than a week, although general fatigue may keep him or her from normal activity levels for weeks to come.

Children with pneumonia can show quite different sets of signs and symptoms. Generally, however, they have had upper-respiratory symptoms such as a runny or stuffy nose for several days; fever and/or chills; a cough; and, occasionally, some chest pain.

Difficulty in breathing leads the child to take fast, shallow breaths; the nostrils might flare outward; the breathing may be accompanied by unusual noises; and, in severe cases, the skin takes on a bluish cast.

ACTION — Once the diagnosis is made and appropriate antibiotics, and possibly an expectorant syrup, are prescribed, most children with pneumonia can be cared for at home. The child should try to rest until 48 hours after the shortness of breath, pain, and fever have gone. Plenty of nutritious liquids can be given, which act to thin secretions and make them easier to cough up. A cool steam vaporizer may be helpful.

If the child suffers from another disease or other diseases, the child's doctor may recommend more stringent measures, including hospitalizing the child to monitor the condition more carefully.

Pneumothorax

A condition in which air escapes from the lungs and out into the immediately surrounding cavity; known more commonly as a collapsed lung.

A pneumothorax can be caused by rupture of the lung or by some penetrating injury to the chest wall. In some newborn babies, especially premature infants on ventilators, weakness of the mid-chest may allow enough tension to build so that pneumothorax develops. However, the hospital staff will be alert to diagnosis and appropriate treatment; complete recovery is the general rule.

Parents should be alert to any sudden and unexplained development of breathlessness and pain or the complaint of a tight feeling in the chest, which worsens when the child breathes deeply. Severe shoulder pain may be experienced on the affected side. In one type of pneumothorax, in which the hole has sealed, symptoms may slowly disappear over a period of a few days.

ACTION — Pneumothorax is not a common disorder among children. Immediate medical attention is required.

Poison Ivy, Poison Oak, and Poison Sumac

An acute inflammation of the skin with blistering, redness, and itching caused by contact with these plants and a sensitivity to the resins in their leaves. It is the same resin in all three plants.

Direct contact is not always necessary to contract this condition; burning leaves that contain the oils of these plants can also spread the poison. Together these three plants create more cases of contact dermatitis than all other causes combined.

Poison ivy usually grows as a low shrub, but when support is available it climbs as a thick vine. The leaves are shiny, three to a stem, and have coarse serrated or toothlike edges. When cold weather approaches, there are clusters of white berries and the leaves change colors. Poison ivy thrives throughout the United States, except for those areas with very dry, hot climates.

Poison sumac, like the other shrubs in its family, may grow into a small tree. The stems are long, with shiny, small leaves arranged along either side and a single leaf at one end. Not nearly as widespread as poison ivy, poison sumac grows primarily in swampy areas.

Poison oak is not a tree, as the name might suggest. It resembles poison ivy, except that the leaves look like oak leaves. The climate along the West Coast of the United States suits the plant well, and it is prevalent in that region.

Contact with the plant or the plant oils causes a reaction anywhere from six hours to six days later, usually in about two days. At first, redness and itching develop. Because contact usually comes from brushing against leaves, the irritation tends to develop in a linear pattern. Blisters soon appear, some of them very large, and the itching becomes intense.

Untreated, and if no secondary infection develops, the rash clears in two to three weeks. If there is a large amount of oil on the skin and the area is scratched, the inflammation can be spread. But contrary to popular belief, fluid from ruptured blisters does not cause any problems.

One very frequently overlooked cause of continual poison ivy, oak, or sumac infections is a household pet that plays in and among these plants and is petted afterwards.

ACTION — Prevention is the best treatment. When children or adults know they might come in contact with underbrush, they should be careful to wear long-sleeved tops, long pants, and high socks so there is less chance of exposure. Parents should know what these plants look like and teach their children which plants to avoid.

Once contact has occurred, the area should be immediately be cleansed with soap (brown soap seems to work best) and water. The old remedy of allowing the brown soap to dry on the skin and then later washing again seems to offer some extra protection: It may absorb the oleoresin (the poisonous oil) before inflammation sets in. The child's clothes should be thoroughly washed or dry-cleaned.

Calamine lotion can reduce the itching of poison ivy-like rashes, but prolonged use may aggravate the problem by accumulating and caking on the skin. Hydrocortisone creams, now available without prescription, may speed healing. Antihistamines may also be useful in relieving the itching.

If the child's doctor or health-care professional suggests the use of moist compresses, parents can prepare them at home by dissolving one packet of a special powder in a pint of cool tap water to make what is known as Burow's solution. In more severe cases that do not respond to home treatment, the child should be seen by a doctor. Short-term use of oral cortisone (for example, prednisone) can provide dramatic relief.

For more information about these conditions, call the toll-free number of Interpro Inc., 800-45-NO-IVY.

Poliomyelitis

A viral disease, also known as infantile paralysis or polio.

Polio may strike in the minor-illness category (with only slight symptoms and full recovery in about three days) or the major-illness category, which may affect the spinal cord and/or brain centers that control breathing and swallowing.

Early symptoms of polio include fever, headache, sore throat, and, sometimes, vomiting. Recovery may follow at this point. If it does not, the child may experience stiffness and a pain in the neck and back, a warning that the disease may be progressing to its more serious, paralytic form.

In paralytic poliomyelitis, fewer than 25 percent of children affected suffer permanent damage to muscles, such as varying forms of paralysis; some 25 percent have mild disabilities; and more than 50 percent recover with no paralysis. However, in children who contract bulbar poliomyelitis, in which breathing and swallowing are severely impaired, the use of artificial aids to respiration is generally required.

The incubation period is from one to two weeks. If polio is even remotely suspected, the child should be put to bed immediately and kept there until medical help — sought on an emergency basis — is available. Activity during the early period of the disease may contribute to the development of paralysis.

ACTION — Unlike parents of one and two generations ago, you need never worry about your children contracting poliomyelitis if you simply take advantage of the effective IMMUNIZATIONS that are now common. Except in people over the age of 16, the original Salk vaccine, given by injection, has now been largely replaced with the Sabin vaccine, which is given by mouth in a liquid form or on a lump of sugar.

Individual doctors differ somewhat in the scheduling of this immunization; some give the first dose when the baby is 2 months old, the second dose at 4 months, a booster dose at 18 months, and another booster with the child nears school-age. It can be given at the same time as DPT (DIPHTHERIA, PERTUSSIS, TETANUS) injections, and parents are urged to consult the child's doctor about arranging for polio immunization.

There are no side effects to the vaccine, and afterward the child may eat and drink as usual and engage in all normal activities. It has been found that out of every 10 million immunizations, only 5 children contract paralysis after they come into contact with the virus. That tiny risk seems far outweighed by the proved benefits of polio immunization for children. However, parents who have not been immunized should avoid contact with an infant who has been given the oral vaccine. It is also possible to acquire the disease by viruses shed in the bowel movements.

Port Wine Stain

See HEMANGIOMA

Postnasal Drip

An increased secretion of mucus, part of which may drain down through the nose, but most of which flows backward and is swallowed.

For the most part, the child is not aware of the process, but if drainage is heavy, especially at night, he or she may experience a choking feeling and cough to try to clear the pooled secretions. Under normal circumstances, air is warmed as it passes through the nose. When children are heavily congested from postnasal drip, they breathe through their mouths and the cooler air irritates the throat.

ACTION — A vaporizer helps keep the drainage loose and flowing, and saltwater nose drops or sprays may help open the airway. Postnasal drip is commonly caused by an ALLERGY, SINUSITIS, or upper-respiratory infection. If a BACTERIAL INFECTION is present, an antibiotic may be needed, so parents are advised to check with the child's doctor or health-care professional.

Prickly Heat

See HEAT RASH

Pyloric Stenosis

A thickening or overgrowth of the pylorus (the muscular ring) at the outlet of the stomach, which prevents normal flow of partially digested food into the intestines.

No one is sure what causes the disorder. It is more common in boys than in girls and occurs more frequently among firstborns. The hereditary influence must not be strong, however, since later-born children in the family have only a slightly greater tendency to have the condition than other children do.

Pyloric stenosis can be congenital (present at birth), but more often it develops over the first month or six weeks of life. Persistent vomiting is a common sign, and it may occur with sufficient force to propel the vomitus for some distance (called projectile vomiting). The baby's distended stomach can actually be observed to make forceful contractions in a futile effort to pass material beyond the blockage.

ACTION — Occasionally doctors try special feedings and the use of an antispasmodic drug. However, surgical correction is very simple and is generally much more successful.

R

Rabies

A viral disease that attacks the nervous system; it is transmitted by bites of infected animals — dogs, cats, foxes, skunks, raccoons, and bats.

Once symptoms appear, rabies is said to be invariably fatal. First symptoms are similar to those of INFLUENZA, followed by progressive irritability, anxiety, insomnia, and pain in the area of the wound. The rabies virus painfully constricts throat muscles if a victim attempts to drink water and swallow it. Heart and breathing muscles are paralyzed, and in the final stages a victim goes into violent convulsions, followed by coma and death.

ACTION — Any animal-bite wound should be cleaned first with soap and water or alcohol and, if possible, be allowed to bleed a little. Then seek immediate medical attention. If possible, the animal should be captured and held for an examination by specialists. With prompt action, effective rabies vaccines can be administered.

Regional Enteritis

A disorder affecting mainly the small intestine, causing the lining to become inflamed, thickened, and less elastic.

Regional enteritis is not a particularly common disease, and it is extremely rare in children under the age of six. Despite the suggestion of a genetic defect, no definitive evidence for a hereditary basis has yet been discovered. Most authorities believe that emotional stress plays a definite role in causing and/or compounding the problem.

Many signs and symptoms may go on as long as three years before telltale signs of intestinal inflammation can be detected by the child's physician. There is also wide variance in symptoms from one child to another — some children experience sharp abdominal cramps or pains during a single, nonrecurrent attack; occasionally, the pains mimic symptoms of acute APPENDICITIS; some children will be nearly incapacitated by the illness, which becomes chronic and may last into adulthood.

Most often the pattern is one of anorexia (diminished appetite), weight loss, nausea, abdominal pain, unexplained fever, and, at times, a hard mass that can be felt in the abdomen. At times the intestinal inflammation may be slight, but the thickness expands to form an INTESTINAL OBSTRUCTION that must be removed surgically. Another complication can occur if the affected area abscesses, walling off part of a perforated section of bowel and creating a fistula (an abnormal passageway to other bowel sections or out to the surface of the body).

To diagnose the condition, the child's doctor may have the youngster swallow a harmless white liquid containing barium. This material is opaque to x-rays so that its progress through the intestinal tract is easy for the examining doctors to follow. Other tests may also be necessary to confirm the diagnosis.

ACTION — If examinations confirm the diagnosis of regional enteritis, various medications may be prescribed, such as antidiarrheals to decrease cramping and diarrhea, hydrocortisone to control inflammation, iron and vitamins to combat anemia or a nutritional deficiency, and antibiotics if infection is contributing to the problem. If medical management fails to correct the disorder, the child's doctor may recommend surgery to remove the diseased sections of intestine. Although this is not a minor operation, it is quite safe in the hands of competent surgeons, and parents need not worry that it will impair their child's normal functioning and/or contribute to the development of other diseases later in life.

Retinitis Pigmentosa

See BLINDNESS

Reye's Syndrome

A potentially fatal disorder that may affect children between the ages of 5 and 15 who have recently been exposed to an acute VIRAL INFECTION *such as* INFLUENZA *or* CHICKEN POX.

Reye's syndrome is characterized by severe disturbances of brain function, increased pressure on the brain, and fatty degeneration of the liver and other internal organs. In very mild cases, only about 20 percent of the cases prove fatal. In children whose illness progresses to convulsive seizures and respiratory arrest, the fatality rate may be over 80 percent. The overall average is slightly higher than 40 percent fatality.

Symptoms include persistent vomiting, high fever, headache, disorientation (lacking conception of time, place, and person), delirium, and fainting, possibly lapsing into coma.

Diagnosis is based on various laboratory findings that include increased ammonia levels in the blood; an abnormally low blood-clotting time; increased brain pressure as determined by examining cerebrospinal fluid; low blood sugar; and many measures of abnormal metabolism. Light-microscopy examination shows an accumulation of fatty deposits in internal organs.

ACTION — Clearly, immediate medical attention and hospitalization are musts. Intravenous fluids are given in an attempt to correct any disturbance in body fluid/electrolyte (essential salts) balance. Intravenous administration of a diuretic (a medication that makes one urinate more frequently) may decrease pressure within the brain. Exchange transfusions (removal and replacement of the child's blood) may be done, and certain drugs, such as citrulline or nicotinic acid, may be used.

More information can be obtained by calling the toll-free number of the National Reye's Syndrome Foundation, 800-233-7393.

Rh Problems

An adverse reaction between a mother's blood and the blood of her unborn baby.

The Rh factor is a special factor in the blood. It gets its name from the first two letters of *Rhesus monkey*, animals with which experimental work was done. If the mother is Rh-negative and the fetus inherits red blood cells of the Rh-positive type from its father, antibodies may be formed. Antibodies are types of body proteins intended to combat foreign substances; in this case, antibodies react against the baby's own red blood cells. These antibodies may cross back and forth across the placental barrier, so that future infants, too, can be affected by the antibodies in the mother's circulation.

Problems may start while the infant is still in the uterus; after birth, ANEMIA and JAUNDICE may occur, as well as seizures, extreme difficulty in breathing, hearing loss, and mental retardation. Some affected infants die shortly after birth; some die while they are still in the uterus.

ACTION — Fortunately, modern medical methods permit early detection of this incompatibility. Both the mother's and the father's blood can be tested so the doctor can be alert to the possibility of Rh problems. The mother can be tested and carefully monitored throughout pregnancy. By a process called *amniocentesis*, material can be withdrawn from inside the birth sac and various analyses can be made to determine how the developing baby is doing.

When an Rh incompatibility exists, the newborn baby is given various blood tests and probably an exchange transfusion of blood. Phototherapy (light therapy) with special fluorescent lights is another treatment used. If appropriate treatment is administered immediately in the newborn period, the baby develops his or her own blood type and no long-term ill effects remain from the Rh incompatibility.

Rheumatic Fever

A joint-inflammation disease that primarily affects children and adolescents, striking children from about age 4 to 18, but mostly between 8 and 15.

Although rheumatic fever is often mild, it is a potentially serious condition. When it is left untreated, it may scar the valves of the heart (rheumatic heart disease), making them too narrow or otherwise unable to perform their normal work.

The exact cause remains unknown, although poor nutrition and cramped living conditions are thought to play some role. Certainly bacteria of the Group A hemolytic *Streptococci* (strep) type are involved, and the disorder generally appears within two to six weeks after a sore throat caused by those germs. It is thought that the disease may represent an allergic reaction to the bacteria's releasing toxins (poisons) into the body, inflaming the delicate linings of the heart and its valves.

After the sore throat or other upper-respiratory infection, symptoms include pain, stiffness, and swelling in one or more of the large joints: shoulder, elbow, wrist, hip, knee, or ankle. Smaller joints are rarely affected. The pain may last only a day or so in a particular joint before it moves on to another. This contrasts with rheumatoid arthritis, in which the pain is more constant in one joint. Other signs and symptoms include fever (which may not be very high), rapid pulse, sweating, and possible pallor (paleness), nosebleeds, and weight loss. Weakness, difficulty breathing, tiredness, and chest pain may occur with heart involvement. In some cases, emotional upset and aimless muscle movements may appear. Sleeping may be difficult if the child is experiencing fairly severe joint pain.

Because many children suffer only mild symptoms, rheumatic fever may go undiagnosed. At best, diagnosis is based primarily on the presence of several symptoms and signs, as well as evidence of a recent strep infection. There is no single test that establishes the disease's presence; some laboratory findings mimic those of other diseases.

In the majority of cases, recovery is complete. In fact, in about half of the patients who are found to have some form of chronic rheumatic heart disease, there is no clear medical history of their having had rheumatic fever.

ACTION — Any child suffering from rheumatic fever should be put to bed at once and kept there until a doctor confirms that it is safe for the child to resume normal or near-normal activities (this may range from two or three weeks to a few months). Judicious bed rest puts less strain on the heart and helps minimize complications. Meals should be light, and liquids should be given generously.

The child's doctor will usually suggest aspirinlike drugs to lower fever and reduce inflammation: He or she may also prescribe antibiotics to wipe out any remaining streptococcal infection and, if necessary, digitalis or other cardiac drugs to treat any heart symptoms.

If the child complains of TINNITUS (ringing in the ears), loss of hearing, or starts to vomit, parents should alert the doctor immediately.

Sometimes hospitalization is recommended during the acute phase, partly to permit more careful monitoring and partly to make sure the child stays in bed.

Rheumatoid Arthritis

See JUVENILE RHEUMATOID ARTHRITIS

Rickettsial Infection

Any infection caused by rickettsia (extremely small parasitic micro-organisms about midway in size between bacteria and viruses).

The rickettsia usually attach themselves to insects and then may be passed on to human beings by insect bites. Such diseases include Rocky Mountain spotted fever, Q fever, and typhus.

Infected children usually show fever and skin rashes. A doctor's diagnostic laboratory tests include measurement of the rise of anti-bodies that specifically fight rickettsial infections.

ACTION — Treatment is by use of a broad-spectrum antibiotic.

Ringworm

A fungus infection of the skin, hair, or nails.

This disorder has nothing to do with worms, but is named after the ringlike lesions produced.

School-age children and adolescents are particularly prone to con-tract *tinea corporis* (ringworm of the body) from floors and shower stalls or benches contaminated with fungi. Pet cats may have facial ringworm lesions that are not noticeable but prove a source of infec-tion to owners who nuzzle their pets.

Tinea capitis (ringworm of the scalp) can be transmitted by the practice of exchanging hats and brushes, by barbers' or hairdressers' instruments, even by leaning against theater seats. Boys are somewhat more susceptible than girls. Tinea capitis is painless, but it causes some patchy hair loss and split hairs, inflammation, and scaling.

ACTION — Treatment for tinea corporis may include scrubbing with skin cleansers such as Betadine; application of antifungal creams; keeping the skin dry; and carefully avoiding any exchange of contami-nated clothing, towels, and linens, which should be boiled or chem-ically sterilized.

Treatment for tinea capitis consists of oral griseofulvin-type antibiotics as well as hygiene measures similar to those described.

Roseola

A viral infection most commonly seen in infants under the age of one year.

The youngster may show a fever as high as 105° F without having many other symptoms. This is generally alarming to parents, but the illness is benign and usually goes away by itself within a week.

The baby may seem droopy when the fever is at its highest, but when it is around 102° or 103° he or she may play and smile. Elevated temperatures usually break after four or five days, and, unlike other viral rashes, it is after the fever breaks that the reddish rash appears, only to fade in about a day or two. The nasal congestion that usually accompanies roseola may occasionally lead to an ear infection.

ACTION — There is no need for concern. However, the parents of other babies that may have come in contact with the infected infant should be alerted to the possibility that their child may have caught the infection.

Roundworm

See ASCARIASIS

Rubella

An acute viral disease, commonly known as German measles.

German measles is a much milder disease of childhood than true MEASLES. It is also much less contagious than "regular" measles, although it, too, is spread by viruses from the nose and throat of an infected person. The incubation period is about two to three weeks.

First signs and symptoms are sore throat, low-grade fever, mild upper-respiratory symptoms, muscular aches and pains, some stiffness of the neck, and some swelling of glands in various parts of the body, particularly below and behind the ears.

The rash, consisting of small, flat, pink spots, may appear first on the face and neck and then spread to the body, particularly the trunk and the limbs.

One attack of German measles usually provides protection for life. It is only in adults that the disorder may be more serious; this is especially so in the case of unimmunized pregnant women, because it can affect the unborn child.

ACTION — Parents should call the doctor for a confirmation of the diagnosis, but rubella is essentially a home-treatable disease. Make sure the child gets plenty of rest, eats lightly, and is given cooling drinks. If itching becomes bothersome, the child can be bathed in cool water. Medicines are generally not needed and should not be given without checking with the child's doctor. An effective IMMUNIZATION against rubella is available and is usually given when the child is 15 months old.

Ruptures

See HERNIA

S

Salmon Patch

See HEMANGIOMA

Scabies

*A red skin rash caused by an allergic reaction to chemicals pro-
duced by small (one-sixtieth of an inch long), insectlike organisms
called* Sarcoptes scabiei *mites that burrow into the skin, causing
bumps, blisters, and red tracks marked by extremely intense
itching.*

Contrary to popular opinion, this infection is not limited to individuals who live in crowded, unsanitary habitats. It is, however,
highly contagious, so if a child is infested, the entire family should be
examined and treated. Bed linens, towels, and clothing should be dry-
cleaned or washed in very hot water, then ironed with a hot iron.

Scabies — sometimes misdiagnosed as ECZEMA, infections, or
drug reactions — usually develops about four to six weeks after exposure. The rash may appear all over the body, but body folds, such as
between the fingers and toes, under the arms, in the groin, or behind
the knee, are particularly susceptible. Infants often show the rash on
their scalp, face, neck, palms, and soles. Scratching causes small
scabs, hence the name scabies, and it can also cause skin scrapes that
become infected by bacteria.

A doctor makes the diagnosis by removing the parasite with a
needle and then examining it under a microscope.

ACTION — Treatment generally consists of cutting the child's nails
short to discourage scratching, use of an antiseptic soap in hot tub
soaks, application of various creams or lotions containing a chemical such as gamma benzene, and, if there is bacterial infection, an

137

antibiotic. The child should be kept home, away from school and/or playmates, until the condition has cleared.

Scarlet Fever

An extremely contagious disease caused by streptococcal infection, which leads to a fine, slightly raised, scarlet-colored rash that begins behind the ears and then spreads rapidly over the entire body.

The incubation period of scarlet fever is from one to five days; the contagious phase usually starts one day after symptoms begin and lasts from two to three weeks if not treated.

The first signs are common to many other illnesses: sore throat, chills, fever, cough, and sometimes nausea and vomiting. The tongue may be covered with a white coating that gradually peels off to show a bright-red strawberry tongue. About a day later the rash usually breaks out, but sometimes it does not appear, and about a week later small round patches of dead skin flake off. A throat culture is necessary to confirm the presences of a strep infection.

ACTION — Modern antibiotic therapy successfully treats this bacterial infection. In addition to the prescribed medications, parents can offer cooling drinks and basically keep the youngster comfortable during the two or three weeks of isolation from other children and family members.

Scoliosis

An unusual, exaggerated, side-to-side or S-shaped curvature of the spine.

Slouching and other signs of poor posture do not cause spinal curvature. In fact, although there is a tendency for the disorder to run in families, doctors can rarely find a specific cause for these curvatures. Apparently a difference in growth rates of the vertebrae (the bones of the spinal columns) causes a twisting or bending of the spine.

Scoliosis seems to affect a number of girls around the time they reach puberty and begin rapid growth. Some studies show that careful screening may uncover cases in younger children. First signs may be a subtle difference in shoulder height or, when the child is viewed from behind, one side of the back is more prominent than the other.

ACTION — Most doctors refer the young person to an orthopedist for an expert opinion. Periodic physical examinations and x-rays may be required. In very mild cases, special exercises may be recommended. In intermediate cases, a brace may be prescribed. These modern braces allow a child to move around and engage in all normal activities, but they may cause a lot of emotional turmoil in young adolescents who are just beginning to care about their appearance. Parents and other family members should be prepared to offer considerable support and understanding.

Only in the most severe cases is surgery recommended — for example, if there is a danger of misshapen arthritis developing or there are chest distortions that might interfere with normal heart and lung function. Prompt professional care may permit the curve to straighten, leaving no deformity.

Seizure Disorders

Episodes of uncontrolled motor activity, usually involving jerking movements, especially of the extremities, and some alteration in consciousness (often, but not necessarily, the loss of it).

All of the following seizure disorders, often called convulsive disorders, involve some disorganization or disruption in the normal flow of nervous impulses coming from the brain.

Epilepsy. If seizures occur before a child is 2, the condition is usually connected to some birth injury, developmental defect, or metabolic disease. In epilepsy affecting children between 2 and 14, no definite cause can be found in more than two thirds of cases. Heredity has long been thought to play a role, but its precise influence has not been fully determined.

Grand mal seizures, also called generalized seizures, are typically preceded by an *aura*: a personal kind of warning system that may be sensed as some vague sensation, image, or thought or as a gut feeling. The aura lasts only about a minute, after which the child usually makes a throat gurgle and then exhibits jerking, twitching convulsions of the whole body. Bladder and bowel control may be lost, drooling may occur, and the child may even turn blue. The seizure itself may last several minutes. Afterward the child is likely to fall into a deep sleep.

In *petit mal seizures*, the child may seem to stare and then twitch, blink, or nod during a 5- to 30-second lapse of consciousness. If undiagnosed, the condition may lead to other problems, because these children are not aware of the lapse of consciousness and, for example, teachers and other children may conclude that they are unintelligent or inattentive.

Diagnosis of epilepsy has been greatly aided by electroencephalogram (EEG) examinations, skull x-rays, lumbar punctures (for examining cerebrospinal fluid), computerized axial tomography (CAT) or magnetic resonance imaging (MRI) scans, and laboratory analyses of serum glucose and calcium levels.

Psychomotor seizures. This condition is characterized by automatic behavior such as lip smacking, running around in circles, or uncontrollable crying or laughing for no perceptible reason. The defect is focused in the temporal lobe of the brain. Extremely careful diagnosis and medical treatment are necessary to control the disorder because, later on, it may lead to violent and potentially dangerous outbursts.

Minor motor convulsions. Infants and toddlers may exhibit seizure episodes in which the head suddenly drops to the chest, the legs come up toward the stomach, and the arms are drawn over the chest. Sometimes small areas of muscles twitch, and sometimes a toddler may seem to be performing some purposeful activity, such as a fancy twisting fall, before parents are aware it is a seizure. Afterward the child may be drowsy or unconscious.

ACTION — Insofar as is possible, children with seizure disorders should be encouraged to lead a normal life. Overprotection may deepen the affected child's sense that he or she is inferior or handicapped. If retardation exists, special-education programs can be helpful. Generally speaking, intelligence is not affected, nor do the seizures necessarily permanently damage the brain.

Frequent medical checkups are a must so that physical disorders such as infections and hormonal imbalances can be corrected and doctors can also determine whether a tumor, an abscess, or the remains of a birth injury may be contributing to the child's problem.

Prescription drugs such as phenytoin and phenobarbital can totally control grand mal seizures in about half the children affected and can greatly reduce them in an additional one third.

Parents and others should learn how to prevent injury by consulting with their doctor about the best course of action for the child.

Normally, clothing around the neck should be loosened, a pillow placed under the neck and the child positioned on his or her side.

NOTE: Parents should understand that the general subject of seizure disorders covers many different kinds of conditions beyond those mentioned here and elsewhere in this book, such as FEVER CONVULSIONS. A more detailed discussion is beyond the scope of this book. The field is so highly specialized that both the child and the parents are best served by consulting appropriate medical specialists who can explain the particular seizure disorder and outline individualized methods of treatment and control.

For more information, call the toll-free number of the Epilepsy Foundation of America, 800-EFA-1000, Monday through Friday, 9 A.M. to 6 P.M. eastern time.

Septicemia

A condition — commonly referred to as blood poisoning — occurring when the bloodstream is invaded by disease-causing bacteria and their toxic by-products.

Symptoms may include the abrupt appearance of high fever, chills, irritability, delirium, extreme lethargy, or even prostration. In severe cases, vascular (blood vessel) shock may ensue, so that blood pressure decreases; the child shows a fast but feeble pulse; the respiratory rate is slowed; paleness or a bluish coloring may occur; skin is sweaty and clammy; and stupor, unconsciousness, or coma can occur. A purplish body rash may develop quickly, which indicates the leakage of blood through small vessels.

ACTION — *This condition should be treated as a medical emergency.* Parents should take the child to a doctor or an emergency facility at once, for children with untreated septicemia can die within hours.

Shin Splints

Intense discomfort of the lower leg(s), usually after heavy exertion, although some individuals may develop pain after a short walk.

Shin splints are uncommon in childhood but may be seen in 5 percent of adolescents, especially among athletes. The pain is thought to come from an inflammation of muscle attachments to the bone. If the muscles are chronically misused, there may be tears of the muscle fibers, and it is this injury that results in the pain and tenderness.

Another defect, called *anterior tibial compartment syndrome*, occurring less frequently than shin splints, develops because the compartment enclosing the lower leg muscles is tighter than it should be. If activity causes sufficient swelling in the lower leg muscles, there may be enough pressure built up to press on arteries that supply the lower leg and foot.

ACTION — For shin splints: Although many cures are offered, the only effective therapy is rest, avoiding running or the activity that caused the pain, until there are no symptoms. This rest period should be at least five to seven days. The next step is avoidance of the activity completely or a change in the child's approach to it. A gradual buildup may help, as may altering the speed, amount of exertion, or even the surface on which any running takes place. Improper footwear may strain lower leg muscles, causing a greater tendency to develop shin splints.

For anterior tibial compartment syndrome: Usually rest relieves the symptoms, but if tingling or weakness of the ankle or foot develops, an urgent medical evaluation is advised. If symptoms of leg pain last longer than 10 to 14 days, a fracture, such as a stress fracture, may be present, and an x-ray is needed for diagnosis.

Shingles

See HERPES ZOSTER

Shock

A type of collapse caused by an extreme deficiency in blood circulation, depriving body tissues and organs of oxygen.

Shock may be caused by injuries and burns, various kinds of POISONING, acute infections, inflammations of internal organs, HEAT STROKE, hemorrhage, ANAPHYLACTIC SHOCK, and other factors that interfere with normal circulation.

A child in shock may show a low body temperature, cold and clammy skin, shallow breathing, a fast but weak pulse, thirst, vomiting, diarrhea, and a general picture of complete prostration.

ACTION — *Shock is a medical emergency.* Treatment may consist of intravenously administered transfusions and solutions, such as glucose; oxygen inhalation; and the use of drugs. A child in shock should immediately be wrapped in a blanket and taken to an emergency facility if an ambulance cannot promptly be dispatched to the home.

Sickle-Cell Disease

Hereditary chronic disease, found primarily in blacks, caused by an abnormality in the hemoglobin, creating a crescent- or sickle-shaped rigid red blood cell.

This disease, afflicting about 10 percent of the American black population (but also occasionally found in people whose ancestry is from the Mediterranean and Middle East regions), is often fatal before age 20 to those most seriously afflicted, and before age 50 for those less afflicted, although a normal life with only occasional setbacks is possible. The sickle-shaped red blood cells have a difficult time passing through the body's smaller blood vessels and often form masses of cells that plug up those vessels. Ironically, the red blood cell distortion has its positive side: It was probably a natural-selection adaptation to life in warm areas, because those with sickle cells are immune to malaria.

The list of symptoms, beyond sickle-cell anemia, is long and grim: abdominal pain, vomiting, joint pain, liver and spleen difficulties leading to painful abdominal bloating, convulsions, ulcers forming around the ankles, kidney disease and failure, headaches, and paralysis.

Sickle-cell disease can grow worse — triggering a dangerous sickle-cell crisis — if the affected child is exposed to very hot or very cold weather, overdoes physical activity, is under stress, or gets an infection. Sudden exposure to cold water can also trigger a crisis; it is believed that the sudden cold increases the thickness of the blood, but a thorough warming after the exposure can prevent problems. Swimming in a heated pool is the wisest way for the child to experience water sports and recreation.

ACTION — Sickle-cell disease has no cure. Treatment is primarily aimed at alleviating symptoms. To that end, the affected child must receive a well-balanced diet, including lots of liquids in an attempt to dilute possible blood cell aggregations; antibiotics may be given to protect the child in case an infection should occur, and corticosteroids may be prescribed to relieve the joint pain.

Parents will almost certainly be urged to get genetic testing and counseling because, as carriers, they may pass sickle-cell disease on to subsequent offspring. If only one parent possesses the abnormal hemoglobin, the chances of the child getting full-blown sickle-cell disease are far less than if both parents have it.

The National Association for Sickle-Cell Diseases offers the following toll-free number to call for information: 800-421-8453.

SIDS

See SUDDEN INFANT DEATH SYNDROME

Sinusitis

Inflammation of the mucous-membrane lining of the sinuses (drainage channels), partly filled with air, in the facial part of the skull.

Infants and very young children have only two pairs of the total of four pairs of sinuses that eventually develop. Therefore, their signs and symptoms may differ from the complaints of older children.

Pain occurs when the inflammation swells narrow openings from the sinus into the nose, so that pressure builds up against the body walls of the sinus. X-rays help identify a blocked sinus, which appears dense because it is filled with fluid rather than air.

Youngsters may show swelling of the skin surrounding the nose and eye. They may seem to have one cold after another, or a cold that never goes away. Older children may complain of headaches, an aching behind the eyes, or tooth pain. Fatigue, a chill, changes in weather, or contact with ALLERGY-stimulating substances may aggravate the condition. Nasal congestions and other symptoms, such as a cough, may resemble the effects of a bad cold; indeed, acute sinusitis frequently follows a cold or other upper-respiratory infection.

ACTION — A doctor's treatment may include prescription nose drops, washing out of the affected sinuses, and, in severe cases, a small incision to allow for proper drainage. An antibiotic will be prescribed if a bacterial infection is present; signs of such an infection include a cough that will not go away, fever, a runny nose, and a persistent postnasal drip. Pus may be present in the nasal discharge.

Parents can help provide relief by applying moist heat compresses; using a vaporizer in the child's room; encouraging the child to drink plenty of liquids, which may help thin secretions; and, if the doctor advises, giving children's doses of aspirinlike painkillers. If the youngster cannot blow his or her own nose, the doctor may instruct parents on how to use a nasal aspirator to suction each nostril gently after nose drops have been given.

Smallpox

An acute, highly contagious, disfiguring, and potentially fatal disease caused by infection with a virus.

Fortunately, smallpox has been conquered by the World Health Organization's worldwide vaccination campaign launched in 1967. Since 1982, the disease has been considered eradicated.

Because of this progress, along with the fact that there has been no case of smallpox reported in the United States or Canada since 1949 and the view of many doctors that the complications from vaccination now outweigh its benefits, children in the United States are no longer required to be vaccinated as a routine precaution. In fact, even children traveling overseas are not vaccinated against smallpox anymore.

Spina Bifida

Congenital condition in which the bony casing around the spinal cord does not develop properly, permitting the spinal cord and meninges to be exposed.

This serious hereditary developmental abnormality occurs during the embryo's first weeks of life in the womb, when the creation of the protective tube around the forming spinal cord does not close completely. After birth, it can be associated with paralysis, deformities, and *hydrocephalus* (commonly known as water on the brain).

Spina bifida occulta is a milder form of the condition in which the neural tube around the spinal cord is not completely fused, but there are no problems or symptoms, and it may go safely undetected for years. It requires no treatment.

However, there are two other, graver types of spina bifida — meningocele, in which the membranes that cover the spinal cord protrude through to the surface of the back, and meningomyelocele, in which both those membranes and parts of the spinal cord and nerve roots are visible.

Some spina bifida babies with severe meningocele or meningomyelocele have brief lives counted in mere hours, while those who do survive longer commonly have mental retardation and limited motor and muscle-control skills.

ACTION — Surgery can aid in relieving many of the possible complications. Parents should seek genetic testing and counseling, for the risk of having another child with the same defect is greater than that in the general population; *amniocentesis* can pick up signs of spina bifida. Professional help should also be sought to aid the parents and any siblings in coping with the familywide problems associated with this condition.

The Spina Bifida Association of America operates a spina bifida information and referral service hot line, offering information about the condition and local chapters in your area. The phone number is 800-621-3141 (301-770-7222 in the Washington, D.C., area).

Spinal Curvature

See SCOLIOSIS

Squint

See STRABISMUS

St. Vitus' Dance

See CHOREA

Steatorrhea

See MALABSORPTION SYNDROME

Still's Disease

See JUVENILE RHEUMATOID ARTHRITIS

Stings

Injuries caused by the mouth parts or stinger and venom of insects.

The stings of bees, wasps, hornets, and yellow jackets cause the greatest number of deaths in children who suffer from ANAPHYLACTIC SHOCK, the most serious form of allergic reaction. Symptoms include extremely severe swelling beyond a joint, wheezing or difficulty in swallowing, fever, and weakness. The child may collapse.

Fortunately, most children are not so sensitive to stings. Unless they are stung inside the mouth or on the tongue (a very serious, potentially life-threatening situation that demands immediate medical care), the normal reaction is simply one of pain and swelling at the site.

ACTION — For nonemergencies: Sometimes the insect leaves its stinger behind, partly embedded in the skin. If this is the case, parents should remove the stinger as soon as possible. Ideally, fine tweezers should be used, but clean fingernails will do. Try to grasp the stinger as close to the skin surface as possible, since squeezing higher up may force any venom still on the stinger into the skin.

Cold compresses may help the discomfort, and a locally applied paste of baking soda mixed with a little water aids in relieving itching and discomfort. Children's dosages of aspirinlike tablets can also be given. Some home remedies may also be of help, including the application of a fresh-cut onion to the stung spot; chemicals in the onion help to reduce pain and swelling.

If increasing pain and redness or swelling develop a day or two afterward, a bacterial infection may have been introduced through the sting hole, and the child should be checked by a doctor.

For emergencies: Treatment calls for an injection of epinephrine (adrenaline), which is present in some emergency kits, or massive doses of antihistamine if the child is able to swallow. Even if parents administer first aid — and especially when they are *not* able to do so — immediate medical attention should be sought for the child; anaphylactic shock can be life threatening.

Once the child is known to be this sensitive to insect bites, parents may wish to discuss the child's undergoing a desensitization procedure. In this procedure, the doctor administers a series of purified venom extracts, which builds the child's resistance to future stings. Recent studies indicate that very few sensitive children, once stung, have as severe a reaction the next time they are stung, thus making the benefit of this costly venom immunotherapy questionable.

Strabismus

A visual disorder, also known as squint or lazy eye, in which both eyes are not directed on the same object at the same time.

Strabismus can occur any time from birth onward. It may show up before the first birthday if muscle imbalance is the cause.

Parents should understand, however, that a number of infants, particularly up to the age of six months, show what is called *pseudostrabismus* (false cross-eyes). It is harmless and requires no treatment, but if it continues after the baby is six months old, it should be checked by a doctor to make sure true strabismus is not involved.

In true strabismus, when children look at an object, only one eye is really seeing it. This is a makeshift, automatic device to prevent double vision, which is intolerably confusing. The youngster simply suppresses the second image. Unless treatment is begun early (say, by the age of five or six), there can be considerable loss of vision, even blindness, in the unused eye. Therefore, young children should be given careful eye examinations that do not rely on the youngster's ability to report what he or she is seeing.

Convergent strabismus is the name for the cross-eyed condition in which both eyes appear to look toward the nose. The crossing can be more pronounced in one eye than in the other, or when the child is looking at a very near or very far object. In another form, both eyes seem to be looking outward. In most instances, however, only one eye is affected.

ACTION — The treatment for strabismus depends on the nature of the squint. If only one eye has been used, patching the overused eye may correct the situation. Special exercises may be assigned for muscle imbalance. Eyedrops and glasses may be prescribed for some deviations that impair vision. Corrective surgery, often done in stages, is generally recommended for children whose cross-eyedness may cause permanent impairment of vision and/or severe emotional problems from realizing that they look odd to other people.

Strawberry Mark

See HEMANGIOMA

Strep Throat

Sore throat (pharyngitis) caused by infection from the Streptococcus *bacterium.*

This sore throat, the symptoms of which are more intense than the run-of-the-mill sore throat, is frequently accompanied by both swollen glands in the neck area and a relatively high fever with headache. It is not unusual to have other frightening symptoms, such as stomach pain and vomiting.

ACTION — The child should be taken to a doctor, who will take a throat culture, examine it to see if Streptococcus bacteria are present (a result that may take a day or two to determine), and then prescribe a regimen of antibiotics, usually for ten days.

See RHEUMATIC FEVER, TONSILLITIS

Sty

A BACTERIAL INFECTION, *usually by the* Staphylococcus *or staph germ, that causes a small abscess of a gland in the eyelids.*

A child may first complain of eye discomfort. Then a small red bump appears along the eyelid near the base of the lashes. Eventually this infection comes to a head and a small center of yellow pus generally drains of its own accord. If it does not, ask the child's doctor if it should be drained professionally.

Even with the best treatment, sties tend to recur; some authorities believe there may be a hereditary basis for them. Sties never suggest a need for eyeglasses.

ACTION — Warm compresses offer some relief. Simply dissolve half a teaspoon of salt in 8 ounces of water and use a folded piece of clean cloth to form a compress that is applied to the child's closed eye for about 20 minutes. Repeat this procedure every hour and a half. An antibiotic ointment or eyedrops may be recommended by the child's doctor.

Sudden Infant Death Syndrome

The sudden and unexplained death of an apparently healthy infant; commonly known as crib death.

Sudden infant death syndrome (SIDS) is the most common cause of death in babies between the ages of two weeks and one year, peaking at three to four months of age, and the second most common cause of death among children as a whole (the first is accidents). In the United States, it strikes approximately 2 infants out of every 1,000 live births, affecting males more often than females, and with the highest incidence among premature babies.

Although immediate autopsy is generally recommended, the results are usually confusing. In only about 15 percent of the cases are there definitive findings, such as some unsuspected central nervous system abnormality, an overwhelming infection, or an undetected abnormality of the heart or blood vessels. Certain changes in the baby's airway, liver, heart, or nervous system may be observed, but none fully explains the death.

Most doctors now believe that SIDS combines many very subtle factors — perhaps some sudden spasm that temporarily interferes with a sleeping infant's breathing, or some other physiological event that cuts off the oxygen supply.

ACTION — When an infant has had an episode of breathing interference and is thus at risk, or when the family has already suffered a loss from SIDS, a monitoring alarm system for home use might be recommended. In some cases its use has led to a baby's survival, but routine monitoring of every infant is not advised.

Families who have suffered through a crib death need very special understanding. They tend to have an almost overwhelming sense of guilt, even when they rationally understand that they are not to blame. Some authorities recommend that professionals visit the home to answer questions about autopsy findings, observe the scene of the crib death, offer reassuring support if parents have had to endure the added stress of a police investigation, and counsel parents both in their grief and with respect to having other children.

A family physician or health-care professional, a local social agency, or members of the International Guild for Infant Survival or the National Foundation for Sudden Infant Death Syndrome can be of help.

There are two toll-free information and referral hot lines concerning sudden infant death syndrome: SIDS National Headquarters, a 24-hour service, reached by dialing 800-638-7437; and the National Foundation for Sudden Infant Death Syndrome at 800-221-SIDS.

Sunburn

Redness, tenderness, or blistering of the skin caused by exposure to the sun.

Infants and young children are especially susceptible to damage by ultraviolet rays from the sun or sunlamps. Even older children, especially if they are fair skinned, should avoid overexposure.

When children are going to be in the sun for a long period of time, say, at the beach, they should apply sunscreen preparations and wear protective clothing except for the briefest excursions into the water. Even an umbrella or other tentlike covering does not prevent the sun's rays from being reflected from the sand, thus causing more of a burn.

A fairly bad sunburn may cause nausea, vomiting, fever and/or chills, and even delirium. Pain increases as the skin reddens and, depending on the extent of skin damage, blisters.

ACTION — Sunburned children should be given lots of fluids. Aloe-containing lotions may help replace lost skin moisture. There are many nonprescription burn ointments, the names of which end in "-caine," that may offer relief from pain. Be cautious about applying them, however, because they may sensitize a child to those medications, which could be helpful in more serious conditions.

If a bad sunburn with extreme reactions occurs, if the burned area is extensive, or if the burn starts to ooze and look infected, take the child to his or her doctor or health-care professional for appropriate treatment, for example, cortisone-type medicines.

Sunken Chest

A congenital (present-at-birth) deformity in which the breastbone and chest are pushed inward in a funnel-like shape.

Sunken chest is more common than PIGEON CHEST and is more likely, in moderate or severe cases, to be associated with heart or lung difficulties, in addition to causing the kinds of psychological difficulties associated with any physical abnormality.

ACTION — If x-ray examination indicates the need for corrective surgery, it should be done during the child's preschool years, after the age of two. If it is decided not to operate, the child should have frequent checkups to make sure there is no interference with chest-cavity functioning and to make sure there is no further cave-in, which sometimes occurs during adolescence and requires surgery at that time.

Compare PIGEON CHEST

Sunstroke

An acute medical emergency, usually caused by excessive exposure to direct sunlight.

Unlike in HEAT STROKE, in sunstroke the skin is red and dry. The child's body feels hot to the touch, breathing is difficult, and there may be a loss of consciousness.

ACTION — The first thing to do is call an ambulance or see that the child is immediately driven to an emergency medical facility. While waiting, or while someone else is driving, the sunstroke victim should be made to lie down out of direct sunlight and with the head and shoulders elevated. The child's entire body should be sponged with cool water, and small sips of cool water may be given if he or she is alert.

Compare HEAT STROKE AND HEAT EXHAUSTION

Swimmer's Ear

Moisture in the ear canal causing inflammation.

Technically termed *otitis externa*, swimmer's ear does not necessarily come from swimming. The inflammation may start in the same way as when skin is exposed to fungi or certain allergic reactions; then bacterial infection sets in, usually by a *Pseudomonas* germ.

Children may complain of pain, itching, swelling, and a possible loss of hearing. A doctor's examination reveals inflammation in the canal, which may already have started to drain outward from the child's ear.

Children who are susceptible to swimmer's ear tend to have recurrent bouts.

ACTION — Treatment may consist of a doctor's careful cleansing of the canal and the possible insertion of a cotton wick so that eardrops can reach all the way through the canal. Antibiotics or corticosteroids are usually prescribed for local application, although they may be given in oral form if the condition has spread. Aspirinlike compounds may be suggested for the relief of pain.

Drops prescribed by the doctor should be kept on hand and used before going to bed on any day the ear canal has gotten wet through swimming or even the everyday activities of showering and getting caught in the rain.

See EAR INFECTIONS

Swollen Glands

Enlargement of the lymph glands.

The lymph glands are like docking points along the channels of the lymph system. They filter and collect invading foreign materials such as bacteria and viruses, proving a first line of defense against disease.

Lymph glands are found throughout the body — in the neck, under the arms, at the elbows, in the groin, behind the knees, and in internal body cavities. They are named according to their location, and they each tend to take care of their own area of the body; for example, neck glands are called cervical glands, and they take care of throat infections and dental abscesses.

Swollen glands are quite common in children. They can last for weeks or even months, and some children seem to have some slight enlargement almost all the time. If the child is thriving and healthy, there is no need for parental concern.

On the other hand, persistent swelling could possibly indicate some serious disorder, such as HODGKIN'S DISEASE, or the development of a tumor at the site of the gland or INFECTIOUS MONONUCLEOSIS.

ACTION — If many groups of nodes show enlargement or if paleness, fatigability, weight loss, fever, or a bleeding problem is present, the child should be examined by a doctor to determine whether some disorder of blood cells might be present.

In general, it is best that a child with swollen glands be checked, even if just for reassurance that his or her swollen lymph nodes are harmless.

T

Tapeworms

A parasitic worm that nests in the human intestines.

Children become infested with tapeworms just as adults do: by eating contaminated and undercooked beef, pork, or fish. The infestation, called *taeniasis*, occurs as a result of swallowing an early form of the parasite, which then develops into a mature adult in the small intestine.

Tapeworms are among the laziest of parasites. They have no mouth and no digestive system; they survive by attaching themselves to their host and soaking up nourishment through their body walls. Tapeworms are formed by a growing chain of separate segments. They have long, flat bodies that resemble a ribbon, and some species in the human intestine may grow more than nine yards (eight meters) long.

Cysticercosis is a condition caused by the eggs of pork tapeworms. Once the eggs hatch in the upper part of the small intestine, they penetrate the mucous walls and are carried to various parts of the body — underlying skin tissue, skeletal muscles, the eye, even the brain.

Unless segments of worms are found in the stool, diagnosis may be elusive, because mature worms usually cause no serious symptoms. However, the psychological effect on children knowing that worms are in their intestines can be devastating. Their presence may produce digestive disturbances such as loss of appetite or a tremendous growth in appetite, as well as abdominal pain and diarrhea.

ACTION — Tapeworms are treated by a carefully combined and medically supervised program of diet, drugs, and purges, which cause the head of the tapeworm to release its hold on the intestinal wall. The parasite is eventually passed out in the stools. With cysticercosis, no specific and wholly effective medical treatment exists, apart from controlling the symptoms.

Tay-Sachs Disease

A genetic disorder leading to the degeneration of brain cells, found primarily in Ashkenazi Jews.

The recessive gene that causes this disease (also known as *amaurotic family idiocy*) is found in approximately 3 percent of Jews with ancestral roots among the European Ashkenazis. Victims, who begin to exhibit symptoms before reaching their first birthday, usually are retarded, become paralyzed and blind, and die before age five.

ACTION — There is no cure for Tay-Sachs disease, and little to do in the way of help except attending to the needs and comforts of the child, whose health progressively worsens. Parents are urged to undergo genetic testing and counseling to determine the realities of having other healthy children.

Tetanus

A frequently fatal disease caused by the Clostridium tetani *bacteria passing into the body through a scratch or wound; since stiffness of the jaw is an early sign, it is commonly known as lockjaw.*

The bacteria live in garden and farm soil, street dust, and even in the intestinal contents of humans and animals, where, in expelled feces, they can continue to live for years. When the wound is extensive — as from a bad cut on rusty metal — or pus-filled, the germs release their toxins, which then circulate through the body.

Tetanus ultimately affects the nervous system and causes a spasm of the facial muscles. Sometimes this spasm is so severe that it creates a fixed, hideous-looking smile; raised eyebrows; and rigid neck muscles. Abdominal and back muscles may also be affected, sometimes causing the entire back to arch forward, and rigidity of the chest wall may interfere with breathing. Convulsions are possible.

ACTION — Tetanus can be prevented by the DPT immunization, which parents should make certain their children receive. Most doctors recommend a periodic booster every five to ten years, depending on the product used. Successful treatment depends on getting the child to a doctor immediately after any wound is sustained by a dirty implement, tool, or piece of rusty metal, or immediately after an injury has been contaminated by soil or other dirt. The child's medical record should indicate whether a booster injection is necessary. Antibiotics may also be given to kill any bacteria that may have entered the wound. If the child is unimmunized, tetanus antitoxin may need to be administered.

Threadworms

See PINWORMS

Thrush

An infection of mucous membranes of the mouth by a yeastlike organism known as Candida albicans; *also known as candidiasis or moniliasis.*

This yeast can usually be found in moist body tissues in the mouth, digestive tract, nostrils, vagina, and other body passages or cavities, and it generally causes no problem unless it begins to grow or multiply at an unusually rapid rate.

Thrush is not uncommon in children. DIAPER RASH also provides a suitable growth place.

In mouth thrush, white patches appear along the inside of the mouth and on the tongue and in the throat.

Young girls may contract vaginal candidiasis (which has nothing to do with having sex), but the risk of yeast growth can be lessened if the child wears loose clothing and cotton panties rather than synthetics, which do not allow for ventilation. In some cases, thrush may develop as a side effect of prolonged antibiotic therapy, which kills certain bacteria that normally restrict an overgrowth of various species of fungi.

ACTION — At the first signs of this fungus infection, the child should be taken to his or her doctor, who will most likely prescribe an antifungal medicine such as nystatin.

See also YEAST INFECTION

Thyroid Disorders

Conditions affecting the functioning of the thyroid gland, which secretes hormones that are necessary for growth and development.

The thyroid gland is located at the base of the neck. It consists of two vertical lobes, one on each side of the trachea (windpipe), connected by a horizontal lobe so that it resembles a fat letter *H*. The thyroid gland regulates the body's metabolism, which is the rate at which the body uses energy. It transforms nutrients and other substances into the various chemicals necessary to maintain life and health.

Hyperthyroidism. A condition in which the thyroid is abnormally overactive and secretes an excess of hormones. Early signs and symptoms include restlessness or nervousness, sweating, rapid heartbeat, and sensitivity to heat. As the disease progresses, the child becomes nervous and jumpy, shows breathlessness, muscle tremors, a staring expression of the eyes, and, despite an increased appetite, loses weight. The disorder more commonly affects school-age children or adolescents, some of whom may show a goiter, which is simply an enlarged thyroid. It occasionally affects newborns, who are extremely irritable and fail to gain weight despite voracious appetites.

Hypothyroidism. A condition in which the thyroid is sluggish and fails to secrete enough hormones. Signs and symptoms vary, depending largely on the child's age. Sometimes the thyroid gland does not develop normally during fetal life.

Congenital (present-at-birth) hypothyroidism can lead to cretinism if left untreated. An affected baby does not grow normally and has an enlarged tongue that eventually may stick out from the mouth, a puffy face, and a snub nose. Mental retardation gradually becomes noticeable, since thyroid hormone is necessary for proper development of the brain. Hypothyroidism is correctable by replacing the missing hormone if treatment is begun before much damage has occurred.

In older children and adolescents, signs and symptoms of hypothyroidism include unusual fatigue, weakness, hoarseness, increased sensitivity to cold, and a pronounced loss of energy and drive. If untreated, the young person may develop *myxedema*, a condition characterized by puffiness of the face and hands, an enlarged tongue that interferes with speech, abnormal weight gain, dry and dull skin and hair, slowed pulse rate, and a general sluggishness of movement.

ACTION — For hyperthyroidism: Treatment usually consists of an antithyroid drug; the possible use of radioactive iodine, which destroys part of the thyroid, thus reducing hormone output; or an operation in which a section of the thyroid gland is removed.

For hypothyroidism: In almost all cases, hypothyroidism can be successfully treated by hormone-replacement therapy, which may have to be continued for life. An adequate intake of iodine should also be maintained to prevent goiter. This can usually be accomplished by using iodized table salt.

Tics

Nervous habits that usually involve a spasmodic, jerking movement of small groups of muscles.

Often facial muscles are involved, as in blinking the eyelids, wrinkling the forehead, grimacing, or twisting the lips, but some children shrug their shoulders or jerk an arm or leg. Sniffing, spitting, coughing, and throat clearing in the absence of clear-cut physical causes may also qualify as tics.

Tics most often develop in the mid-school-age period, around the age of ten, but they can occur in both younger and older children. Tension seems to be the most prominent cause. This may require parents to reexamine day-to-day living patterns in the home; readjust their own expectations (achievement anxiety may lead children to develop tics); and perhaps help the child explore ways in which he or she might profitably cut back on strain-inducing, competitive activities. The child can be reminded gently of the tic when it occurs and how it may be upsetting to people who watch it, but the young person should never be scolded or punished.

ACTION — Most tics disappear of their own accord as the child outgrows the tension point. Few tics have any neurological basis. However, parents — and the child too — may want to seek professional help to make sure that a disorder such as TOURETTE'S SYNDROME is not present, as well as for some guidance in sorting out reasons for the tic and how it might be managed.

Tinea

See RINGWORM

Tinnitus

The sensation of a buzzing, ringing, or roaring sound in the ear.

Tinnitus may result from a mild head injury or blow to the ear, from the presence of water or too much wax in the outer canal, or from overexposure to extremely high noise levels. Tinnitus may be associated with EAR INFECTIONS, damage to nerves supplying the ear, or, on rare occasions, some psychiatric disorder.

Many young children these days have Walkman-type radios or tape players, which they listen to using headsets or earphones. Eighty-five decibels is the limit the Occupational Safety and Health Administration has set for what a human can stand without risking damage over the course of an eight-hour workday. One hundred decibels for one hour puts a person in risk of permanent hearing damage. Loud music on either high- or low-quality earphones can produce sounds of 110 decibels or higher. That is why high-volume music on earphones is considered a prime cause of hearing loss in youngsters and adolescents, with ringing ears a primary result.

ACTION — If a child complains repeatedly of hearing abnormal sounds, he or she should be examined by a physician or health-care professional. Parents also need to be reminded that tinnitus sometimes results from use or overuse of a number of prescription and nonprescription drugs. If this happens, notify the child's doctor immediately so that the dosage can be adjusted or another product can be substituted.

Toeing In

Walking with the toes pointed toward the center of the body.

Toeing in is very common in early childhood, but in most circumstances it is outgrown before the child reaches school age.

While the baby is in the uterus, the legs and feet are folded across the lower part of the body. It takes several months for the tendency to this position to change, and it does not happen fully until the infant stands and walks around.

In some cases, toeing in may be caused by tibial torsion (rotation of the shinbone) or femoral torsion (rotation of the thigh bone), or by metatarsus adductus (a curved or hooked foot).

ACTION — Most cases of tibial torsion correct themselves, although severe cases may warrant the use of special night braces. Femoral torsion is also generally outgrown; braces and special shoes do not seem to help. A hooked foot may be corrected by special exercises that press the toes outward. As this condition is often noticed when a baby is only a few weeks old, parents may be instructed by the child's doctor how to perform these stretching exercises on the infant's foot. In severe cases, a cast or brace may be applied.

Toeing Out

Walking with the toes pointed away from the center of the body.

The normal gait of human beings is one in which there is a slight toeing out. Babies do this to a pronounced degree. However, with continued weight bearing, the feet rotate inward until a more usual position is attained.

Concern should arise only if there seems to be no change after a few months, if the deformity is severe enough that a toddler has difficulty walking, or if the youngster appears to be walking on the inner sides of the feet.

ACTION — Serious, fixed rotations may require special orthopedic procedures; doctors or other health-care professionals can determine this during early, routine examinations.

Tongue-tie

A short attachment between the underside of the tongue and the floor of the mouth; not to be confused with STUTTERING or stammering.

In true tongue-tie there is rarely enough restriction to cause any difficulty with either feeding or speech development.

ACTION — Unless the tip of the tongue curls downward to a marked degree and cannot be extended out to the gums, no treatment is indicated. If a really significant shortening exists, the child's doctor may recommend a plastic-surgery revision rather than just snipping the tissue.

Tonsillitis

An inflammation of the tonsils, caused by a viral or bacterial infection.

The tonsils and adenoids are similar to lymph nodes found throughout the body. They are believed to act as germ traps. Children's tonsils normally vary in size and they continue to gradually diminish in size. In very young children, the tonsils often appear so large that they nearly touch. However, unless they are also very red or have white or yellow patches on the surface, they are probably not infected.

The child with infected tonsils shows signs of throat pain, difficulty in swallowing, and fever. Peak incidence tends to occur when children are between two and six years old, and some youngsters may have three or four attacks each year.

Adenoids are situated high on the back wall of the pharynx (throat), behind the opening from the nose. Adenoids, too, are most prominent in young children; before adolescence they disappear altogether. When children's adenoids become grossly enlarged, they often make it difficult for a child to breathe through the nose. POSTNASAL DRIP, coughing, and SNORING are frequent results of enlarged adenoids, as is a blockage of the eustachian tubes leading to the ears, which can contribute to EAR INFECTIONS.

ACTION — Once the particular germs causing the tonsillitis have been identified, the child's doctor may prescribe antibiotics. Allowing the child to suck on crushed ice may relieve the pain.

In current medical practice, removing the tonsils is generally not recommended unless they become chronically infected or abscessed or the enlargement is extreme. If the adenoids contribute to serious impairments such as chronic ear infections, removal may be recommended. Snoring and impaired sleep (obstructive sleep apnea), as well as a failure to grow at the same rate as other children the same age, are also good reasons to have the surgery performed.

In the hands of a competent surgeon, the operation is extremely simple and sometimes may be performed as a short-stay procedure. Nonetheless, parents should carefully prepare their child by explaining what will be done, how the child might feel afterward (throat irritation is common), and, to the extent the child can understand, why the operation must be done.

Tourette's Syndrome

A condition manifested by facial and vocal tics, usually starting in childhood, lessening during adolescence, then flaring up again during adult life in the form of generalized jerking movements of the body.

Tourette's syndrome, named for a turn-of-the-century French physician, is generally assumed to be hereditary and associated with some disorder of the brain that does not affect intellect, but the exact cause is unknown. Signs and symptoms include TICS (involuntary blinking and muscular twitching), grimaces, general jerking movements of the arms and shoulders, banding of the arms, grunting sounds, barking noises, shouting, and, in about half of those afflicted, compulsive swearing or the use of obscene language. It tends to affect three times as many boys as girls, and only 30 percent of those affected require treatment — the other 70 percent have symptoms too mild to treat. There is no known cure.

ACTION — Control of the symptoms can often be achieved through using the drug haloperidol (Haldol), although some sufferers claim improvement from behavior and dietary therapies.

More information may be obtained by calling the toll-free number of the Tourette Syndrome Association, 800-237-0717.

Tuberculosis

An infectious bacterial disease caused by the tubercle bacillus.

There has been a dramatic decline in childhood tuberculosis (TB) over the past half century or more; there are now probably fewer than 3 new cases each year per every 100,000 children in the United States.

Some newborn babies may contract TB if their mothers have active — unhealed and contagious — pulmonary (lung) tuberculosis. Drug treatment is usually given, although frequent blood, liver, and ear tests are recommended because of some questions concerning the safe use of such drugs in young babies. Some doctors prefer to use the BCG (Bacillus Calmette-Guerin) vaccine to prevent TB in high-risk infants, that is, those born to a mother with active tuberculosis.

The widespread use of pasteurized milk and laws that require the testing of cattle have reduced the incidence bovine-transmitted TB, caused when the bacilli enter the bloodstream through the mouth. The disease is usually transmitted through contact with a person who has active tuberculosis. Once it is inactive, the disease is no longer contagious.

What is termed *primary tuberculosis* is the site where the infection is initially located, usually the lung. The infected site heals within a couple of months. Eventually a chest x-ray may show nothing more than a small calcified area where the TB node healed. Generally, neither the parents nor the child knows TB was ever present, since there are rarely significant symptoms.

At times, however, that area of primary focus breaks down and reinfection occurs. The child or adolescent looks quite ill, and fever, night sweats, difficult breathing, cough, weight loss, and malaise (a generalized feeling of being unwell) are present.

Two special, but fairly rare, kinds of TB should be mentioned. *Miliary tuberculosis* occurs when there is a massive invasion of the bloodstream by TB germs. Children affected have anorexia (loss of appetite), fail to thrive, and run a fever; medical examination reveals a swollen liver and spleen, and x-rays show widespread mottling of the lungs. In *tubercular meningitis*, the infection spreads to the central nervous system and causes fever, irritability, stiff neck, seizures, and perhaps coma. Immediate medical treatment is necessary.

ACTION — Treatment includes isoniazid (a potent antituberculosis drug), an appropriate antibiotic, and a healthy diet with vitamin supplements. Once the child feels better, resting is no longer considered necessary, nor is the isolation that was once required. After the disease is under control, the child should return to school. If necessary, the child's doctor, who uses periodic x-rays to check gradual disappearance of the disease, can explain to school personnel that the condition is no longer contagious.

Many schools and other facilities give routine screening tests for TB. Small amounts of tuberculin are injected beneath the skin. A positive reaction produces a red area of inflammation, which indicates the child may have had TB in the past. A sputum culture and chest x-ray are recommended as follow-ups to a positive skin test.

U

Undescended Testicle

The failure of one or both of the testes (testicles) to assume their normal location within the scrotal sac.

In fetal life, the testicles remain high in the abdomen, being connected to several structures, including the vas deferens, a tube that transports sperm (the male reproductive cells). By the time of birth, the testicles usually slip down through a canal in the groin and into the scrotum.

Sometimes this descent does not occur, especially in prematurely born infants, so one or both testes remain in the abdominal cavity. In a condition known as *retractile testis*, a testis may reach the scrotal sac but then be pulled back up into the abdominal cavity. A doctor can manipulate the gland back down into the scrotal sac without surgery.

ACTION — Although hormonal treatment has been and sometimes still is used, results have not always been promising. Generally speaking, if both testes remain in the abdominal cavity after puberty, the boy remains sterile whether or not surgery is performed. The operation shows a good success rate and requires only a brief hospitalization of two or three days. Ideally, any repair should be done before school age to avoid exposing the boy to peers who are apt to mock his visible abnormality.

Urinary-Tract Infection

See CYSTITIS, KIDNEY INFECTIONS AND DISEASES.

Urticaria

See HIVES

V

Vaginal Itching

See VAGINITIS

Vaginitis

Inflammation of the vagina, often accompanied by intense itching.

Symptoms of vaginitis may include an increased urge to urinate, pain on urination, and a vaginal discharge that may contain pus or blood and that, in severe cases, is foul-smelling and extremely copious.

In adolescent girls who are sexually active, gonorrhea may be a cause. However, there are many other possible causes: BACTERIAL INFECTION from nonvenereal germs; fungal infections (YEAST INFECTIONS); protozoal infections such as trichomoniasis; irritation from the insertion of foreign bodies or from chemicals used in douches; infestation with worms; and, although rare, vitamin deficiency. Medical evaluation is necessary to determine the exact cause or causes so that appropriate treatment can be prescribed.

ACTION — The temporary application of warm, not hot, saltwater (made with one teaspoon salt to one pint of water) gauze dressings may offer some relief from the swelling and itching. Warm tub baths may also help. Girls should avoid bubble baths, which inflame the area even more, and avoid wearing panties made of synthetic materials, which impede ventilation.

Viral Infections

Any disease or disorder caused by infection with a specific virus.

Viruses are a wide group of microorganisms much smaller than bacteria. Viruses reproduce only within living cells, to which they attach as parasites.

165

ACTION — In general, viruses are not affected by antibiotics or other drugs, although antibiotics are sometimes prescribed in an effort to combat a secondary infection superimposed by bacteria. As yet, there is no protection against any of the more than 100 viruses responsible for the COMMON COLD.

Prevention, however, is possible for viral diseases such as MEASLES and INFLUENZA, for which effective immunization exists.

Warts

A viral skin infection.

Warts can be any size; they can be smooth and only slightly raised, or rough and considerably elevated. The hands, elbows, fingers, and occasionally the soles of the feet, where they are called plantar warts, are the most commonly affected areas.

Warts may take as long as six months to develop. One fourth disappear within six months after they appear; a full two thirds are gone within two years. Picking at the warts may spread the virus to other areas.

ACTION — Warts need medical treatment only if they are painful, spread rapidly, or enlarge enough to be cosmetically disturbing. They may be painted with special chemicals such as a strong acid, frozen off, or removed surgically.

Wasp Stings

See STINGS

Whooping Cough

See PERTUSSIS

Y

Yeast Infection

Candidiasis *or moniliasis, the technical terms for yeast infections, cause certain microorganisms to grow, especially* Candida albicans, *which is responsible for* THRUSH *and a form of* VAGINITIS.

Yeast infection occurs when the fungus grows and multiplies at an abnormal rate. This situation may occur as a result of lowered body resistance, such as when bacteria that normally perform protective functions are destroyed by antibiotics given to control some other infection; or when some body change creates a climate more favorable to the growth of the fungus.

ACTION — Vaginal yeast infections usually produce a thick, cheesy discharge, which should be carefully cleansed away from the child's genital area. Frequent baths in tepid water and wearing cotton underwear that allows for ventilation help. However, the only really effective treatment depends on prompt medical evaluation and diagnosis so that an appropriate fungus-fighting drug, such as nystatin, can be prescribed.

Yellow Jacket Stings

See STINGS

COMPLAINTS, CONCERNS, AND PROBLEMS

A

Abdominal Bloating

The abdomen is that part of the body situated between the chest and the pelvis (lowest part of the trunk). The abdominal cavity contains the stomach, small intestine, large intestine (the colon), liver, pancreas, spleen, kidneys, and bladder; in females it also contains the uterus and ovaries.

A newborn infant's abdomen normally appears larger than one would expect in relationship to other body parts. When a baby is lying down, the abdomen has a full, rounded appearance. As the youngster begins to stand and walk, the fullness becomes even more noticeable. At around the age of two years, as the abdominal muscles strengthen, the toddler's profile becomes flatter.

Some swelling or bloating may occur when a child is overfed or has swallowed an excessive amount of air. The problem is relieved when the child vomits or defecates. More persistent bloating may indicate that the child is not absorbing nutrients properly, a condition generally associated with poor weight gain. Chronic CONSTIPATION may also cause the abdomen to look full and rounded. If persistent bloating is observed, medical attention should be sought.

Remember: All young babies normally have protruding bellies that sometimes give them the appearance of a miniature Santa Claus. Parents should keep in mind that it is *rapid abdominal distension* that sounds the alarm. A prompt medical examination is in order whenever swelling of the abdomen exceeds the quantity or quality usually considered normal for infants and toddlers. Other disorders not mentioned here combine to make abdominal bloating a serious sign that — except in an obvious instance of overeating or swallowing too much air — should never be ignored or downplayed.

See CANCER, HERNIA, INTESTINAL OBSTRUCTION

Abdominal Pain

One of the most common complaints in childhood is that of abdominal pain. The abdominal cavity contains the stomach, small and large intestines, kidneys, bladder, liver, pancreas, spleen, and, in females, the reproductive organs. The first sign of an underlying problem affecting any of these organs may be abdominal pain. Although the causes are often minor — hunger, overeating, gas, fatigue, or overexertion — a parent must always be alert to the possibility of a significant medical condition.

The nature and apparent location of the discomfort are important diagnostic clues for the physician. For example, the pain may be sharp and highly localized in one area of the abdomen, or it may be experienced as a dull and poorly localized sensation. It may be fairly constant or tend to come and go, in which case it is called cramping or intermittent.

The age of the child is another important factor in determining possible causes of abdominal pain. When a child is old enough to describe the nature of abdominal discomfort, it is much easier for the parents, and the physician, to determine what might be wrong — or at least to attempt to identify the most likely cause. In children too young to verbalize their discomfort, the diagnosis may be more difficult. Infants generally communicate their distress by crying. Distressed infants commonly cry in a way that sensitive listeners can quickly distinguish from a "feed-me" cry.

Psychosomatic factors can also cause abdominal pain in children. A fear of school, social pressures, or anxiety can cause pain that is experienced as quite real. Children need to have this pain recognized and dealt with either by reassurance and supportive measures or through professional consultation.

Parents should note any associated signs or symptoms and describe them as accurately as they can:

- Is there vomiting or diarrhea?
- Has there been any fever?
- Are urinary symptoms present, such as burning or greater frequency?
- Is there a relationship to meals or feeding?
- When did the child last have a bowel movement?
- If the pain comes and goes, is there any apparent pattern in timing and intensity?

- Does anything seem to offer relief?
- Is the pain related to any signs of undue nervousness or agitation?
- If this is a recurrent bout, has there been a change in appetite or a loss of weight since the last episode?
- Is there a history of injury to the abdomen?

The answers to such questions will help a doctor assess the situation.

Fortunately, most cases of abdominal pain in children are not serious. However, if the pain comes on suddenly or persists for more than an hour or two, seek a physician's help, especially if the pain is accompanied by vomiting. Do *not* give the child solid foods until advised to do so by the child's doctor. If the child is thirsty, he or she may, with the doctor's permission, be given small sips of water or other cool drinks. But if these fluids are not retained, call the doctor again. *Above all, children with acute abdominal pain should never be given a laxative or cathartic.* In certain conditions, including APPEN-DICITIS, such medicines could cause intestinal damage and further pain.

See APPENDICITIS, CYSTITIS, GASTROENTERITIS, INTESTINAL OBSTRUC-TION, INTUSSUSCEPTION, KIDNEY INFECTIONS AND DISEASES, MECKEL'S DI-VERTICULUM, PERITONITIS

Addiction, Warning Signs of

It seems a bit bizarre for parents with a martini in one hand and a cigarette in the other to approach their preteen or teenage child and announce, "Don't you ever fool around with marijuana!"

In fact, parents may have even more to do with substance abuse than just setting a bad example; it is very likely that some genetic "addictive personality" component might be handed down from generation to generation. But just because such a component is there does not mean that it has to be acted on, and it may not be without the right (that is, the wrong) environment.

Adolescents frequently experiment with drugs because of peer pressure, rebelliousness, or, particularly with alcohol, because they think this is grown-up behavior. Parental intervention just might exacerbate the situation.

Substance abuse to the point of addiction necessitates that a professional counselor enter the scene. Dependency might be suggested by:

- School truancy and lowered academic performance
- Seeming lack of initiative
- Inappropriate spending of money
- Unusual nasal congestion
- Changes in appetite
- Glassy eyes
- Marked changes in behavior, such as hyperactivity or fatigue

Direct confrontation does not work. Parents should check with an appropriately trained professional — a physician or other health-care professional, a counselor, a social agency or drug-counseling center, or a member of the clergy — who is experienced in this field.

This is a complex issue, mixing the personal and the political, the psychological and the criminal, and it can set parent against child in ways that may take a long time to heal. It is keenly important that the right steps be known — and taken. No brief entry in a book crowded with assistance for other conditions and concerns can do it justice. To get more complete help and information — and support — parents may want to call one of the following toll-free numbers: Alcohol Abuse Emergency 24-Hour Hot Line, 800-252-6465; Alcohol and Drug Helpline, 800-821-4357; Just Dial No, 800-USA-1-MAN; Just Say No Foundation, 800-258-2766; National Cocaine Hot Line, 800-COCAINE; National Drug Information Referral Line, 800-662-HELP; National Parents' Resource of the Institute for Drug Education, 800-677-7433.

Aggressive Behavior

Many theories have been advanced to explain how a pattern of aggressive behavior — in which a child displays a strong tendency toward fighting, instigating disorder, and infringing on the rights of others — may develop. For example, bad behavior may lead to punishment, which may lead to anger and aggressive feelings, which may lead to bad behavior. Violence on television and aggressive models such as a parent or older sibling have also been suggested as causes.

Perhaps of most importance to the concerned parent is the realization that behavior that may be entirely appropriate at the age of 2 may be totally inappropriate at the age of 8 or 12. When the child is showing behavior that is out of the ordinary for same-age peers or for certain social situations, parents should not block it from their minds in the mistaken belief that it is just a phase. Or, in the event of a teacher's complaints that a child is unruly or provocative, parents should try not to fall into the trap of believing that their child is right and the outsider is wrong.

If a careful and honest review of the home atmosphere fails to reveal causes or contributors that are easily remedied, the situation should be discussed at once with the child's pediatrician or a professional counselor. The sooner a repair process begins, the better the likelihood of a successful outcome.

Appetite, Changes in

An almost constant concern to most parents is what and how much their children eat. Books on nutrition are widely available, and many of them offer some reasonable guidelines.

Normal eating patterns vary during a child's growing years. During the first year of life, an infant gains weight and grows in length at a pace never to be achieved again. By one year the birth weight is tripled and the baby has grown about ten inches. Because of the demands posed by this growth, a baby eats what seems like an incredible amount of milk and solids. At the end of the first year, however, the growth rate slows noticeably and does not pick up much until adolescence.

In the preschool years, a child's weight gain is about 5 pounds a year; the increase in height, about 2½ inches. During this time, children's appetites decrease considerably. A demand for fluids remains, but a toddler may go for extended periods of time — even for a few days — without wanting much in the way of solids. This can be frustrating to parents, and if they are not careful they may unwittingly contribute to future feeding difficulties for the child. Undue concern on the parents' part can force children to become obstinate about eating; then a vicious cycle develops.

Although nutritious foods should be offered on a regular basis, parents should not always demand that they be eaten. Similarly, junk foods, sweets, and carbonated beverages should be avoided as a routine, but an occasional treat is acceptable and may also convince a child that meals are okay too.

Parents who get upset when their children do not eat may benefit from an interesting experiment. Fill your plate with the following: a one-pound patty of ground beef, four cups of french fries, and three cups of some vegetable you are not particularly fond of. Then fill a one-quart pitcher three-quarters full of milk. Now, despite your busy afternoon and the fact that you may not feel very hungry, sit down and quietly eat this dinner. Since you weigh about three or four times what your child does, these portions may equal what you put on a child's plate. The moral of the story: Be careful to serve children portions they can handle.

Also, listen to what your children tell you. They just may know what is good for them. Remember the old "ideal" breakfast of eggs and two or three strips of bacon? These foods happen to contain high amounts of cholesterol, saturated fat, and salt, not to mention potentially dangerous preservatives in most bacon.

Keep in mind that meals should be pleasant, restful times with an air of ease; a time to take care of self and a time to talk about the day's activities. Any demand for another kind of performance — that is, eating — makes the period stressful for the child.

Remember, too, that when children reach their next period of growth spurt — adolescence — they will probably munch their way through everything that is not nailed to the floor.

In general, parents should not worry about changes in appetite unless the child shows noticeable weight loss or gain, fever, marked irritability, or gastrointestinal symptoms, any of which may signal a possible disease state.

Attention Span, Short

As most parents have already observed, the very young toddler tends to move quickly from one activity to another. By the time youngsters are ready for school, they can usually work through the beginning, middle, and end of an activity, and the impulsiveness characteristic of the toddler stage has been curbed by many socialization influences.

Children with short attention spans — who have an inability to maintain concentration on some given task or thought — most often bring to school a set of behaviors that is really characteristic of an earlier stage of development. They may be seen as misbehaving and be disciplined because of it; since they really cannot control their efforts, such children tend to become angry and thus even less amenable to learning.

Psychological testing may be helpful in defining the problem and suggesting methods of coping with it. In some instances, medication may improve the attention span by lessening hyperactivity. Professional help is required and should be sought early to prevent the child from growing up with a poor self-image and from being regarded as a troublemaker.

See ATTENTION-DEFICIT DISORDERS

B

Backache

The spine is actually a series of joints similar to those elsewhere in the human body, even though most people do not regard the backbone as such. Alongside this system of bones and ligaments (fibers that connect bone to bone) are elongated muscle masses that allow movement and also provide stability. An injury to the bone or ligaments, or a severe pull on these back muscles, causes a spasm. The spasm acts to prevent further movement by the simple mechanism of causing pain. Children may twist their backs while playing, cause strain by lifting objects too heavy for them, or sustain a direct injury to the back, perhaps by falling. The painful discomfort caused is usually aggravated by movement and may be partially relieved by having the child lie on a firm, flat surface.

Back pain can signal structural deformities of the legs, especially if one leg is shorter than the other. Although unusual in childhood but occasionally seen in late adolescence, back discomfort associated with pain in the buttocks or the legs may occur because of a protruding intervertebral disc (slipped disc), and special x-rays are required to make this diagnosis.

When the pain strikes suddenly and there is no known injury, several possibilities must be considered. Back discomfort can occur in flu-type illnesses; it is usually connected with a generalized achy feeling. In the case of KIDNEY INFECTION, the pain is usually off to one side or the other rather than in the center of the back. Also, cysts, tumors, and infections may develop in the bones of the spine itself.

In a child who appears to be ill, rapidly developing lower back pain may be a sign of MENINGITIS, especially when there is also fever and vomiting. Not infrequently, neck stiffness and pain are also present.

If signs of meningitis or other serious conditions accompany the back pain, immediate medical attention is mandatory. Treatment of back strains generally consists of rest, taking aspirin as often as the directions say is acceptable for children, and the use of cold packs, being careful not to cause damage to the skin. Sleeping on a rug or pad on the floor may also help. Rest should be continued until walking or engaging in other movements does not cause pain. If these measures do not bring a pattern of steady improvement, medical evaluation is necessary to determine if a more serious problem exists.

Bad Breath

Medically known as *halitosis*, breath odor in children can usually be traced to poor dental hygiene or tooth decay. Children should be taught to brush and floss so that a buildup of plaque does not occur. Dental plaque houses bacteria that can cause decay, further adding to bad breath.

Other unpleasant mouth odors can occur with disease. For example, an acute or chronic infection of the tonsils or back part of the child's nose may result in bad breath. DIABETES MELLITUS and other disturbances in metabolism can cause the breath to have the odor of acetone, which smells like an open bottle of fingernail-polish remover. On rare occasions, breath may smell like ammonia or urine if a child's kidneys are not functioning properly; but this is a late sign and by that time so many other symptoms will have appeared that the child will undoubtedly be in treatment, so this type of bad breath may never develop.

Balding

See HAIR, LOSS AND THINNING

Bed-Wetting

When a young child has not yet reached the stage of fairly constant daytime control, *enuresis* (the medical term for bed-wetting) is to be expected. Many normal healthy children continue to wet the bed at night long after they have achieved good daytime control. A parent need have little concern unless the nighttime bed-wetting persists much beyond the age of five years — although even then an occasional mishap should probably be overlooked.

Bed-wetting seems to be more common among boys. This may reflect a high degree of physical and emotional activity that, in turn, induces such deep sleep that the sphincter muscle that controls the bladder loosens and urine flows.

A hidden urinary-tract infection can cause enuresis, and this may be especially true for girls. Although such infections as well as other medical conditions (a SEIZURE DISORDER, certain hormonal imbalances, DIABETES MELLITUS) can cause bed-wetting, parents should be relieved to know that most cases stem from less serious problems. Also, many of these situations can be effectively managed by a combination of supportive reassurance and simple teaching techniques.

Helping children gain nighttime control involves some retraining. Often all that is needed is restricting fluid intake after dinner — limiting children to no more than a few ounces of water — and awakening them to get up and urinate just before parents go to bed.

Older children may benefit by setting an alarm to go off just before the time they generally wet the bed. A degree of responsibility and self-sufficiency can be fostered if these children are provided with dry bedclothes and pajamas and told that they should not disturb their parents during the night.

Some electronic devices are available commercially. One alarm sounds whenever the bed is wet. After a period of several weeks the child is conditioned to respond to bladder fullness before the alarm goes off. Another device hooks directly to the child's pajamas. Its alarm is a buzzer that rests on the child's pillow and awakens only him or her, not the entire household.

Certain methods of bladder training may be suggested by the child's doctor. Parents may be asked to help teach the child during waking hours to retain urine for as long as possible and then record the volume of urine passed. Another alternative is medication, although this is generally not done if the child is under the age of six years, and parents must ensure that dose and timing instructions are followed to the letter.

Emotional difficulties must, of course, be considered. The pendulum has swung away from its old direction — that is, the belief that bed-wetting is always a symptom of severe psychological disturbance. But stress, anxiety, fear of parental rejection, envy of a younger sibling's bed-wetting "privileges," and other factors can play a definite role in a child's continued bed-wetting or regression to that behavior once he or she has outgrown it.

For almost all children, nighttime wetting is an embarrassing and demeaning affair. Parents who become so frustrated that they punish, tease, or reprimand only compound the problem. Supportive reassurance works far better than punishment, and parents who take an active part in applying retraining techniques can encourage cooperation on the child's part.

If the situation is not alleviated by some of the techniques mentioned here, professional psychological evaluation is in order. This is especially so when other signs of immaturity, such as temper tantrums or late thumb sucking, are present. Sometimes hypnosis is effective, but any such treatment should be undertaken only by qualified professionals once a psychological evaluation suggests a deep-seated emotional problem and a medical evaluation has eliminated the possibility of some organic defect or infectious disease.

Behavior Changes in Teenagers

It is a basic characteristic of human beings to have variations in mood and behavior. Everyone has good days and bad days. The reasons for these changes are frequently multiple, but even singly they may be very complex. If we do not feel well physically, if the weather is bad, or if our plans go awry, we may react negatively to those around us. In the same way, when everything goes well, we tend to react positively.

What emerges even with the changes, however, is a pattern of behavior that is fairly consistent and readily observed by others. A child's emerging personality pattern is discernible to parents. Moods can be sensed, and some of the child's reactions are often predictable. It is normal for adolescence to be accompanied by wide mood swings that make it more difficult for parents to monitor the flow of feelings. But alert parents can usually judge how life is going for their child. Being a good observer is a crucial part of parenting. Development of a sense of how a child reacts to stress, for example, helps parents provide support when it is needed. Similarly, parents can develop a sense of when to bring a subject up for discussion; that is, they know when their interest may be perceived as invasive and when the child is silently asking them to help by sympathetically listening and talking.

Gradual behavior changes toward more social responsibility indicate that the child is maturing. For instance, a teenager who has been driving too fast begins to slow down — an indication of accepting adult-level responsibility.

If, on the other hand, parents note accumulating negativity in their adolescent's behavior, it is a sign that the child may be having difficulty handling something stressful. Irritability and FATIGABILITY are important signals parents should be aware of. When causes are not obvious or if the unhappiness is persistent, close attention must be paid. It is important for parents to remember that their own negative reactions to a child's negative behavior only aggravate the situation. Try to develop a tone of support. If such efforts do not succeed, seek the advice of the child's physician.

Very abrupt changes in an adolescent's behavior, whether negative or positive, require special consideration. A teenager who has been previously withdrawn and acting depressed may become relaxed, even jovial, when he or she reaches a decision to attempt suicide. Deceptively, a teenager's mood may lighten tremendously after deciding to run away from home. These quick changes in mood occur when a person who has been wrestling with a problem for a long time suddenly sees a solution, no matter how dramatic, or even life threatening, that solution may be.

Behavior changes may also occur when a teenager is experimenting with, or regularly using, drugs.

Gradual positive changes are healthy. Negative changes should cause concern. Sudden and unexplained behavior changes, either positive or negative, should be scrutinized carefully.

Blood in the Stools

Sometimes called rectal bleeding, blood in the stools generally indicates that either an irritation or a structural abnormality exists somewhere along the digestive tract.

Unlike ANAL FISSURES, rectal bleeding requires a thorough medical evaluation. An exception to this rule may be made when children have consumed beets, certain fruit, artificially colored drinks, or other foods that cause a red or purple discoloration in a child's bowel movement that is not really blood. If this is the case, and the situation does not recur until the next purplish-red meal, parents need not be alarmed. But if there is any doubt, a simple chemical test done in a doctor's office can confirm the nature of the liquid or solid discoloration.

Note the amount, the frequency, and the color of the bleeding so that an accurate report can be made to the doctor. Blood coming from high in the digestive tract — that is, from the mouth, throat, esophagus, or stomach — has a black, thick, sticky appearance: the so-called tarry stool. This dark coloration is caused by stomach acid and other chemicals that play a role in digestion. Blood swallowed from a nosebleed may also produce tarry stools.

Blood-streaked mucus may show up in the bowel movements of children — especially young infants — who have acute GASTROEN-TERITIS, a common viral illness that inflames the stomach and intestines. In these instances, there is not a great deal of blood and the bleeding subsides when the child stops vomiting and suffering diarrhea.

Bloody diarrhea may occur with certain bacterial infections of the intestines such as salmonella or shigella. Usually the child also has a fever over 102° F. Most commonly, these disorders clear up by themselves, although occasionally antibiotic therapy may be necessary. Bloody diarrhea also frequently accompanies inflammatory intestinal diseases such as REGIONAL ENTERITIS and COLITIS. In severe cases, abdominal cramping, weight loss, and FATIGABILITY from ANEMIA are prominent features.

Bright red blood mixed with a bowel movement can occur from a MECKEL'S DIVERTICULUM or, more often, as the result of an intestinal polyp (a small growth). These little growths are most often found in the lower section of the intestinal tract when the physician uses an instrument called a sigmoidoscope to inspect them and sometimes take a biopsy specimen. Children's polyps are very rarely malignant, and the doctor may choose not even to remove them. However, especially if they are large, they may cause a rather copious amount of bright red rectal bleeding, which may be alarming to the parent and to the child. However disconcerting the situation, it is rarely a dangerous one. Only when there is family history of multiple polyps, and the child shows the same tendency, need any extensive surgery be undertaken.

Occasionally bleeding from the intestinal tract may be so slow that no blood is noticed in the child's stools. The diagnosis will usually be made while a physician is searching for the cause of ANEMIA. INTUS-SUSCEPTION may also cause rectal bleeding that shows up as a thick, stringy bowel movement called currant jelly stool.

As noted, blood in the stool may occur in a number of illnesses that are not serious, or the "blood" may be nothing more than coloring from some food or drink. But, on occasion, there may be blood loss that warrants specific therapy, or an illness or structural abnormality that needs prompt medical attention. So when parents first suspect rectal bleeding, they should certainly consult with a doctor.

Blood in the Urine

Discoloration of the urine is technically known as *hematuria.* If the child's urine appears reddish or tea colored, parents should first carefully review what the youngster has had to eat or drink in the previous 12 to 24 hours. For example, beets or artificial food colorings may cause an unusual color in the urine. However, if parents are at all uncertain, they should check with a doctor. A simple chemical test done in the doctor's office will clarify whether blood is actually present.

Blood in the urine, which generally also contains pus cells the doctor can note by microscope, may occur in urinary-tract infections. Parents may begin to suspect this condition if the child makes frequent trips to the bathroom and complains of discomfort on urination. The treatment generally consists of oral antibiotics.

Children with nephritis (kidney inflammation) tend to pass a dark red or brown urine. In one form of this disease, acute glomerulonephritis, infrequent urination may be a symptom, and the child shows swelling of body parts, especially the eyelids and, in males, the scrotum. Once the diagnosis is made, treatment most likely includes the restriction of fluids. Generally speaking, the kidneys heal in a period of weeks and the child suffers no long-term harm.

Injuries may also cause bloody urine, as can happen if there is a tear in kidney tissue caused by a direct blow to either of the kidney areas. So-called ammonia burns — inflamed areas at the tip of the penis — may cause small amounts of bleeding that seem to be coming with urination. Frequent application of a protective cream allows these so-called burns to heal, and no further treatment is needed. An inflammation of tissues around the vaginal opening may be responsible for blood that appears to accompany the flow of urine in girls. In both boys and girls, direct injury to the genitals may cause bright red bleeding. A medical examination is necessary to ensure that no serious tears are present.

On occasion, small amounts of blood in the urine may not be noticed at all, but they may be detected when tests are done as part of a routine physical examination. When this occurs, other signs and symptoms of illness, as well as family history, will be used by the physician to reach a diagnosis.

Since there are any number of conditions that may be associated with blood in the urine, parents should not delay seeking medical advice if their children show any evidence of such bleeding.

See KIDNEY INFECTIONS AND DISEASES

Blood in the Vomitus

The appearance of bright red or dark blood in the fluids a child vomits frequently arises from an irritation at the back of the nose or throat. On occasion, prolonged or particularly forceful retching tears the small blood vessels in the esophagus (the swallowing channel), which produces tiny patches of blood in the child's vomitus.

Before the parent becomes unduly concerned, it is a good idea to review what the child has eaten or drunk over the previous several hours. Red dyes used in food and drink colorings, as well as certain foods themselves, may be the real source of what appears to be blood. If there is any doubt, a simple chemical test done in a doctor's office or an emergency room will settle the question.

Parents may also want to carefully monitor their children when they take seemingly harmless drugs such as aspirin. Aspirin can irritate the stomach and cause bleeding that may be vomited.

When a child suffers a nosebleed, fairly large amounts of blood may be swallowed. If the blood remains in the stomach for even a short period of time, it may be regurgitated as a dark-colored material resembling coffee grounds. The coffee-grounds consistency and dark brown or black color may also characterize blood vomited when the child has a peptic ulcer or some other problem involving the esophagus or stomach. If more than a tablespoon of such vomitus appears, urgent medical evaluation is necessary. Coffee-grounds vomitus is a classic sign of CANCER of the stomach, although parents should be reassured that children are very rarely afflicted with that disorder.

If there is internal bleeding that is brisk, the vomitus is bright red. Here, too, parents should seek immediate medical attention.

Certain caustic poisons, if eaten or drunk, cause severe burning of the upper intestinal tract, resulting in the vomiting of blood.

In general, blood in the vomit can signal an extremely serious condition, and, unless food coloring is suspected, it is wise to seek medical assistance as quickly as possible. If there is any reason to suspect the child has ingested caustic poisons, call for immediate emergency assistance and also contact the nearest poison-control center for advice about first-aid procedures. Parents should keep this number beside the telephone at all times; there is a space at the front of this book to write your local number. You can get the number from Appendix III (see p. 305).

Blood Pressure, High

Blood pressure tends to vary according to a person's body position, level of activity, and other factors, but a school-age child's systolic (top) and diastolic (bottom) blood pressure measurements should probably never exceed 100/80 or 110/80.

Up until and including about the age of 4, an average reading is 85/60. Then, for a while, the top figure increases approximately 5 points with every 2 years of age added. The increase then slows until the adolescent is about 16.

See HYPERTENSION; BLOOD PRESSURE in Appendix I: Norms and Values

Blood Transfusions

Surgery may occasionally require the replacement of blood lost during the operation. But today, with the panic caused by incidents of AIDS being transmitted through blood transfusions some years back, there is fear and even reluctance among many parents to let their children receive blood. Even though hospital industry experts and the American Red Cross attest that the risk of getting AIDS-tainted blood is low to practically nonexistent because of newer and better screening methods, the fear is unabated.

There are two ways to allay the concern. The first is to have a parent, sibling, or close relative with the same blood type as the child — and known to be AIDS free — give blood to the child. This can be arranged ahead of time when the surgery is of the elective, non-emergency kind.

The second way to assure that children avoid getting somebody else's blood during surgery is to make sure they get their own. Autologous blood donation is a method by which a person, knowing that he or she is going to have surgery in the near future, donates his or her own blood to be stored specifically for his or her operation. When the surgery is at hand, the blood is removed from cold storage and made ready if the situation warrants it.

Check with the child's doctor or surgeon to see if autologous blood giving is a possibility, or discuss it with a representative of the local American Red Cross. Keep in mind that such blood storing would need to be initiated many weeks, even months, ahead of the surgery date.

See AIDS

Blurred Vision

This partial or total blurring can result from eye injuries, eye infections, certain diseases or structural defects of the eye or optic nerve, or as a side effect from prescription or over-the-counter drugs.

Because it is essential that the underlying cause be determined and, if possible, treated and corrected, parents should not attempt to treat such a condition themselves. If a child complains of blurred vision or a younger, nonverbal youngster seems to have trouble focusing on objects, he or she should immediately be taken to a physician or eye specialist, who can determine what is wrong.

See also FARSIGHTEDNESS, NEARSIGHTEDNESS

Body Temperature, Abnormal

The heat of the human body is measured in degrees Fahrenheit (° F) or degrees Celsius or Centigrade (° C). The average body temperature, taken by mouth with a clinical thermometer, is 98.6° F or 37° C. However, this figure may vary slightly from one individual to another, or at different times during the day, or when extreme activity or noticeable change in air temperature causes variations that can be considered normal. In other words, within limits, there is no "right" temperature.

This variation in children's body temperature is noticeable in newborn babies, especially if they are premature or sick. Newborns can be affected not only by the temperature of the air but also by humidity, air flow, and the temperature of surfaces they are in contact with, for example, bedclothes or a mattress.

Until a child is old enough to be relied upon to hold a thermometer under his or her tongue, a youngster's temperature should be taken rectally or under the armpit. The parent should keep in mind, however, that a rectal temperature can be expected to read about 1° F higher than one taken orally; an axillary (under-the-armpit) temperature may read about 1° to 2° F lower than on an oral thermometer.

Parents whose children customarily show slight variations in body temperatures without showing any signs of illness need not be unduly alarmed. They may wish to keep track of these variations and perhaps tie them to certain environmental or activity factors before consulting their physician or health-care professional about whether the child should be professionally examined.

See also FEVER, HYPOTHERMIA; TEMPERATURE in Appendix I: Norms and Values

Bottle-Feeding, End to

Many parents wonder and worry about when to take their children off the bottle and teach them to use a cup, either a regular cup or a "sippy cup" with a small spout. These parents are often concerned that the child might be on the bottle too long, or that they are taking the child off the bottle too quickly — either the child is slow or the parents are fast.

It is difficult to make a hard-and-fast rule about this — children move ahead at different paces. Generally, though, if the child can drink from a cup, and does so some of the time, then a bottle is no longer necessary. But some youngsters want to hang on to bottle use until age three or slightly beyond. This is not wrong but, perhaps, slightly past time. The National Parenting Center recommends:

- Weaning a child off the bottle gradually
- Stopping him or her from carrying the bottle around or taking it to bed
- Eliminating time-of-day bottle feedings in this order: midday, afternoon, morning, and bedtime, and for the last bottle slowly reduce the amount of liquid in the bottle daily over the course of a week

Some children will put up a fuss about losing their bottles, which may have become objects of security, identity, and even control over the parents. Some parents use techniques such as trading the bottle at a toy store for a toy the child really wants, or wrapping the bottle up and pretending to mail it to a figure the child believes in, such as Santa Claus or the tooth fairy. Others simply, and effectively, tell the child that the bottles have been given away. A little crying may occur, but it is over quickly, and the bottle will soon be forgotten. If a nighttime bottle is given, only water should be used (not milk or sweet liquids) to avoid the tooth decay that sometimes occurs.

Bowel Movement, Abnormal

It is important for parents to understand their child's usual bowel movement pattern so they can notice any change that may signal the need to consult a physician.

The bowel movements of a newborn baby may be green and sticky for the first few days. This is caused by meconium (a substance created in the intestinal tract while the baby is in the uterus). Transitional stools — a mixture of green and yellow — then follow.

During the first few months of life, babies tend to have as many as five or six yellow, "seedy," watery bowel movements a day. This pattern is especially true for breast-fed infants, although it is also seen in babies taking formulas; it simply means that the young baby is efficiently using all the milk being taken in, so that there is little left but water to excrete.

On the other hand, infants may reabsorb all the water and fluids from their diet; when this happens, the baby may go for a day or two without dirtying a diaper. Sometimes an infant may shift between these two patterns. However, if three days go by without a bowel movement, stimulating the rectum with a lubricated thermometer or a glycerin suppository may be required to cause a movement. If this does not work, *do not give the infant a laxative of any sort.* Consult the baby's doctor at once. Although the condition is rare, sometimes the last portion of a very young baby's intestinal tract does not move correctly and the infant would go on without evacuating unless surgically treated.

As the infant grows and begins eating solid food, a more definite bowel movement pattern is established. Usually one to three yellow-to-brown movements are passed each day. The stools are pasty to firm, and the odor and color depend on what the child has eaten.

When toilet training is achieved, and especially by the time a child starts school, the usual pattern is one or two soft but well-formed bowel movements a day. Parents should remember, however, that variations may occur when there are diet changes — for example, high intake of fluids or eating too much or too little fiber.

Parents are frequently concerned when babies and youngsters show signs of discomfort as they have a bowel movement. Bright red faces, grunting noises, and occasional crying are common signs. If the stool appears normal once it is passed, parents need not be concerned. This straining process is nature's way of helping the baby increase the abdominal pressure that is necessary to pass a normal bowel movement. When the stools appear hard and pelletlike, parents can give the child a commercial stool softener — a tablespoonful a day, in either milk or water — to help loosen the consistency of the movement. This quantity can be increased to two tablespoonfuls a day if the problem persists. When the child's stools are soft and easily passed, taper off the softener or consult a doctor or health-care professional for advice about whether to continue, stop, or switch to some other method if necessary.

Changes parents may notice include:

- Diarrhea, which could signal the presence of an acute infection
- Bloody diarrhea, especially when abdominal pain is present, which might indicate REGIONAL ENTERITIS or COLITIS
- CONSTIPATION, especially when it is chronic, which should generally be evaluated by a doctor before any therapy is started

Laxatives should *never* be given to a child. In addition to irritating the intestinal tract, they may cause a dependency called the laxative habit, which leads to the use of stronger and stronger medications. In some cases, such as APPENDICITIS, the use of laxatives can cause extreme harm.

BLOOD IN THE STOOLS, ABDOMINAL BLOATING, VOMITING, and black, tarry movements are some signs that indicate the presence of a significant disease; the child needs to be examined by a physician. Very light-colored or white stools may be found in HEPATITIS. Slimy green bowel movements with mucus in them may indicate swallowed drainage from some upper-respiratory disorder, or possibly some disease affecting the intestinal tract. Foul-smelling fatty stools that float on the toilet water may be found in CYSTIC FIBROSIS and in MALABSORPTION SYNDROME. Children who have been placed on a liquid diet may, after two or three days, expel green watery movements called starvation stools.

When parents cannot readily tie children's changed bowel movement patterns to diet, fluid intake, or minor infections such as the COMMON COLD, they should consult a physician.

See also FECAL SOILING

Breast-Feeding, Problems with

Much has been written and broadcast about the whys, hows, and wherefores of breast-feeding, and the La Leche League can and will answer most of your questions (ask your doctor or health-care professional for the phone number of the local chapter in your area). A few points to keep in mind concerning the baby's health are:

- Many mothers do not know if they are doing it right. They worry that the baby is not receiving enough milk, and this fear is compounded if the child falls below what is considered the norms for his or her age group. In general, if the baby is alert and content, has regular bowel movements, is going through about a half-dozen diapers a day, and is gaining weight, then he or she would seem to be thriving on the breast-feeding regimen. If the baby is not, the mother should discuss with the doctor whether she should cease breast-feeding altogether, or whether a combination of formula and mother's milk will be satisfactory.

- Mothers may take their success or failure at breast-feeding personally, as if they are somehow lesser human beings for producing small amounts of milk compared to the allegedly copious amounts their female friends, relatives, and fellow nursing mothers make available to their infants. Breast-feeding is not a competition, and what is normal for one woman is not normal for another. The election for the post of SuperMom will not be won or lost on liquid measurement.

- Mother's nipples can become sore if the baby latches on tightly and often. Salves and moisturizers can help, but be aware that some moisturizers and lotions contain ingredients that the baby may be allergic or sensitive to; for instance, if the child is allergic to wool, it would be unwise to apply lanolin to chapped nipples.

- Women who want to breast-feed but are having problems nursing can get help not only through the La Leche League but also from certified lactation consultants who may work with or for the hospital where the baby was born.

- Breast-fed babies are prone to suffer from JAUNDICE more than formula-fed infants, but if blood tests show no liver problems and the doctor seems unconcerned, there is no need to stop breast-feeding. Just keep alert for any worsening of the jaundice, and try to give the baby a lot of natural outdoor light (or the doctor may want to provide ultraviolet light treatments for the child). The jaundice should disappear in a week or so.

Breast Size, Changes in

Female breasts begin to develop at puberty, although this may occur earlier and should cause no concern unless other secondary sexual characteristics also make an early appearance, in which case medical attention should be sought.

Some teenage girls are worried by one of two concerns: Their breasts seem to be either too small or too large. Occasionally, if a girl is unduly preoccupied by what she perceives as underdevelopment or overdevelopment, she may wish to discuss the matter with a physician or psychologist. More often than not, some reassurance from her mother and her own gradual realization that breasts are by no means the sole key to attractiveness enable the female adolescent to overcome her shyness and concern.

Breath Holding

In this type of behavior, an infant or young child — usually in the toddler stage — consciously holds his or her breath. This usually occurs as a response to frustration, an expression of anger, or a kind of testing of new-found abilities, much as TEMPER TANTRUMS are.

The color of the youngster's face goes from red to purple to blue. The event may proceed to a point where the child does, in fact, stop breathing for a moment or two, usually no longer than one minute, at which time there may be a loss of consciousness. However, should this occur, nature's protective mechanism comes into play and the child starts breathing again spontaneously — just as we breathe when we are asleep because parts of our brain and respiratory system work without our conscious control.

If the episode is a long one, twitching movements or even convulsions are possible. However frightening — even terrifying — the event may be for the parent, there are no harmful or long-term effects from a breath-holding spell.

An old recommendation to parents was that they ignore such outbursts and perhaps even leave the room. This seems unwise. Children in this state ought to be observed. If the color changes progress to white or ashen and the child is not breathing, mouth-to-mouth resuscitation should be started. In more extreme cases, if the heartbeat or pulse is absent, full cardiopulmonary resuscitation should be undertaken. One should not begin cardiac massage unless the heart has stopped. A good rule for parents to follow is: Simply observe the child to make sure nothing unusual is happening; otherwise, let the episode continue through its stages, giving it no special attention and never intervening to try to stop it by shaking or holding the child.

Children should not be allowed to acquire the habit of breath holding because they sense it is an effective emotional tool useful to defy parental control. At the earliest opportunity, discuss the problem with the child's doctor or health-care professional. Perhaps special tests such as an electroencephalogram may be warranted to make sure there is no neurological or other medical component present. If parents can determine what kinds of events seem to kick off such behavior, perhaps they can be avoided. But parents should not give children their own way just to avoid the frustration that culminates in a breath-holding spell. A physician's or psychologist's advice may be helpful to parents confronted by the dilemma of what to do and what not to do. Fortunately, in most instances, toddlers outgrow this behavior when they learn that there are more socially acceptable ways to express their frustration.

Bruising

Many parents become concerned about the ease with which their children bruise. Black-and-blue marks on the legs are fairly common as a result of bumps and falls suffered during normal play and physical activity. However, if the child goes to bed with no apparent marks and gets up with bruises, especially on the back or chest, a medical difficulty involving spontaneous bleeding may be present. This situation warrants immediate medical attention.

For minor bruises, parents can administer first aid by intermittently applying cold wet compresses, an ice bag, or freshwater ice. Saltwater ice should be avoided because the temperature of the slush is low enough to cause further tissue damage. The child should rest the injured part so that blood flow is not increased by activity. After about 24 hours, a heating pad or hot wet dressings can be used. If the bruise does not improve in two days, or if it continues to increase in size, medical attention is necessary.

Burns and Scalds

Children are very prone to getting burned as they experiment with their own increased mobility, investigate interesting-looking things they may want to touch, or, quite literally, play with fire.

Burns are traditionally classified according to the degree of tissue damage:

- First-degree burns involve only the epidermis (the outer layer of skin), and are limited to reddening.
- Second-degree burns involve both the epidermis and the dermis (the inner layer of skin), and they blister.
- Third-degree burns involve not only the epidermis and dermis, but also the tissues below the skin. The skin itself may be charred black, or it may appear pale white.

Third-degree burns are a medical emergency. All third-degree burns and any burn that affects more than 10 percent of a child's body surface demand immediate hospitalization. *SHOULD YOUR CHILD BE BURNED IN THIS WAY, CALL AN AMBULANCE OR TAKE THE CHILD TO A HOSPITAL EMERGENCY ROOM WITHOUT DELAY.*

As a good rule, parents should not attempt to home treat any burns except minor ones that cover only a small area and quite clearly are no worse than second degree.

Currently accepted first-aid treatment for first- and second-degree burns is to apply very cold wet compresses or freshwater, *not* saltwater, ice packs. The affected area may also be immersed in or placed under running cold water, although the latter may further damage skin if the stream is too fast and forceful. These measures help relieve pain and they may also minimize tissue destruction or the formation of blisters. It is best not to apply any ointment unless the child's physician advises otherwise. Minor burns are also best left open to the air rather than being covered by any bandage or dressing.

The old remedies of greasy materials such as butter or lard should never be used. The doctor may, however, recommend application of some water-soluble antiseptic that also has anesthetic (painkilling) effects.

Again, parents should keep in mind that severe burns or scalds, especially when they involve large areas of a child's body, can be life threatening. Fluid loss, BACTERIAL INFECTION, and many other factors come into play.

C

Chest Pains

In most instances, chest pain in children and adolescents is perfectly harmless.

Adolescents are especially prone to recurrent episodes of sharp pain in the front of the chest, perhaps with a sensation of shortness of breath. There is no known cause for this; it is probably related to growth.

Children's chest pain is often related to overeating, which causes INDIGESTION, or muscular strain from playing hard.

Unless the pain is prolonged, persistent, severe, or seems to limit activity, parents need not be too concerned.

See also PLEURISY, PNEUMONIA, PNEUMOTHORAX

Compare ABDOMINAL PAIN

Chills

Chills typically precede many fevers children get, and they may occur when youngsters are contracting INFLUENZA, PNEUMONIA, or other infectious diseases. However, a chill is not always a symptom of infection; it may occur when a child has been given fever-reducing medications, including aspirin. Sometimes chills accompany an allergic reaction, a transfusion reaction, or the presence of some malignancy. Repeated chills are common in blood-carried infections caused by bacteria (bacteremia), in acute infections of the kidney, when the child has ENDOCARDITIS (an inflammation of the membrane that lines the heart and its valves), and with certain abscesses.

Children experiencing chills should be made as comfortable as possible in a warm, but not stuffy, room, and perhaps by adding an extra blanket. Hot drinks may be soothing. Parents should take the child's temperature as soon as possible, repeating this about every 20 minutes until 20 minutes after the chill subsides. If the parent decides to seek medical advice, this temperature record, as well as information about the duration and severity of the chill, is helpful to the physician or health-care professional.

Choking

The aspiration of a foreign body is a common hazard and one of the greatest causes of home accidental death in children under five years old. Any foreign body in the upper airway is an immediate threat to life and requires urgent removal.

If the child can speak or breathe and is coughing, any maneuvers are dangerous and unnecessary. If the choking child is unable to breathe or make a sound, is turning blue because of lack of oxygen, or has become unconscious due to lack of oxygen to the brain, measures must be taken immediately. Finger probing of the mouth should be attempted only if the foreign body is visible; even then, doing so risks pushing the object even further into the throat, lodging it more securely.

Today, the widely accepted method of dislodging food or other items from the upper airways is the *Heimlich maneuver*, which uses the air blocked up and remaining in the lungs to propel the stuck food or object out through the mouth.

According to Henry J. Heimlich, M.D., this is the proper way to perform the Heimlich maneuver:

From a standing position:

1. Stand behind the choking victim.
2. Wrap your arms around the victim's waist.
3. Make a fist, placing the thumb *slightly* above the navel (belly button) but *below* the rib cage.
4. Grab your fist with your other hand and press into the victim's abdomen with a *quick upward thrust.*
5. If necessary — if the object has not been dislodged and the victim is still choking — repeat this procedure, several times if need be.

The Heimlich maneuver can be performed on a choking victim who is seated (stand behind the chair and do the same procedure as if he or she were standing) or lying on his or her back.

According to the American Heart Association and the American

Academy of Pediatrics, a combination of back blows and chest thrusts is recommended for choking infants:

1. Straddle the infant over your arm, with the head lower than the trunk. Firmly hold the jaw to support the head.
2. Forcefully apply four back blows with the heel of your hand between the infant's shoulder blades.
3. After the back blows have been delivered, place your free hand on the infant's back so the infant is between your two hands, one supporting the back, the other the neck, jaw, and chest.
4. While continuing to support the head and neck, place the infant face up on your thigh and apply four chest thrusts.

Circumcision

Except as a matter of religious ritual, circumcision — the surgical removal of the prepuce (the skin fold covering the head of the penis) — is now the object of considerable controversy. Advocates stress ease of hygiene, avoidance of inflammation, and less risk of contracting venereal disease; some research tends to indicate that circumcised males have fewer urinary-tract infections. The American Academy of Pediatrics claims there is no evidence to support routine performance of the operation.

When circumcision is performed, it is usually done shortly after birth. No anesthetic is used, the operation usually takes no more than 15 minutes, and the risks involved are minimal. Either a metal or plastic bell is used to control the bleeding while the skin is removed. In some techniques, a plastic ring is left on to provide pressure so that no bleeding occurs and to help promote healing. This plastic device should fall off by the eighth day; if it does not, parents should contact the baby's doctor.

Care of a circumcision is relatively simple. For the first few days after the operation there may be a thick yellow material that adheres as healing takes place. Merely keep the area well-cleaned with soap and water and apply petroleum jelly to prevent irritation from diapers or other underclothing. If there is any untoward swelling, bleeding, or apparent difficulty in urinating, call the doctor.

When an uncircumcised baby is bathed, the foreskin should be brought all the way back so that the head of the penis can be properly cleaned. On occasion an extra fold of skin will remain. Just like the foreskin, this fold of skin should be retracted for washing. As the little boy grows, he can be taught to do this himself.

Colic

Colic is a collection of symptoms and signs usually confined to very young infants. It does no permanent harm and almost always disappears of its own accord by the time the baby is three or four months old. However, until that time the irritability of an infant in apparent pain may put enormous physical and psychological stress on the parents, who often need to be reassured that they are not guilty of anything, that they are not being bad parents, and that the infant is not seriously ill and will recover. Sometimes a sympathetic physician or other health-care professional will suggest that the colicky baby be placed in the hands of a competent baby-sitter while the distraught parents enjoy a couple of hours having dinner out or at some distracting show or musical event.

The cause of colic is unknown, although some authorities believe it may be connected to one or more of the following: swallowing air, overfeeding, intestinal allergy, poor digestion in the form of excessive fermentation of carbohydrates in the intestines, and, on rare occasion, some emotional upset.

It is easy to understand parents' concern. The infant with colic may cry incessantly, apparently from ABDOMINAL PAIN. The abdomen is usually distended and tense, and colicky infants typically draw up their legs against the abdomen and clench their hands. An attack, often occurring at about the same time each day, usually in the late afternoon or evening, may last from two to ten minutes, only to be followed by another one a very short time later. Sometimes an attack will subside only when the child is completely exhausted.

Parents can often help relieve colic attacks by placing the baby stomach-down across their knees or against the shoulder, or in the crib on a pillow, and gently rubbing the baby's back. Sometimes placing a hot-water bottle filled with lukewarm water against the infant's stomach helps. Rectal stimulation with a lubricated thermometer or a glycerin suppository may be effective because it has been noticed that colicky babies seem to be relieved when they have a bowel movement or pass gas. Giving the infant simethicone drops to break up any gas bubbles may also help.

If the doctor suspects a MILK ALLERGY, a switch to soybean milk may be suggested. If the infant is being breast-fed, the mother may be asked to eliminate certain foods from her diet, such as cabbage and onions. In especially severe cases, a physician may prescribe a sedative for the child.

If attacks of colic are associated with vomiting or abdominal bloating, it is particularly important to have the child examined by a doctor to determine if something more serious, such as INTESTINAL OBSTRUCTION, may be causing the infant's pain.

Compulsive Behavior

Children with compulsive behavior — in which there is repetition of a particular physical act or acts over a long period of time — may, for example, be able to go to sleep only after every pair of socks in the bedroom is carefully rolled and placed in rows in a dresser drawer. A classic example is the need to wash one's hands 20 or 30 times a day when there is no reason to do so.

Often such actions are performed as substitutes for thinking about frightening, tension-causing feelings of anger or resentment, or as a means of avoiding some underlying conflict. The compulsive behavior, being ritualistic, affords the child some magic way of warding off thoughts and feelings he or she senses it is best to keep on an unconscious level. If these acts are severe enough to interfere with normal functioning, or if they seem to be preventing a child from developing new social skills normal for school-age youngsters, parents are advised to seek help from a physician or psychologist.

On the other hand, normal school-age children frequently develop temporary behavior patterns that seem ritualistic and obsessive. For example, they may avoid stepping on cracks in the sidewalk; tell endless jokes that seem nonsensical to adults; make noises with their tongues; annoy adults by counting telephone poles or reading signs out loud during automobile trips; cross their eyes for the fun of it; or, sometimes, even develop little facial TICS (repetitive muscle spasms) that distort their features and alarm concerned parents. For the most part, these behaviors reflect youngsters' attempts to master their own bodies and put the environment into some ordered relationship.

Parents should grin and bear it and not rush the child off for counseling or a neurological examination unless the behavior persists unduly or unless a young adolescent suddenly exhibits compulsive behavior that is quite different in nature and intensity from his or her usual patterns.

Constipation

In infants, constipation — the difficult and too-infrequent passage of dry, hard bowel movements — may result from drinking too much milk. Diet is also an important factor in youngsters and older children, especially if they eat too little fiber or roughage.

Sometimes children repeatedly fail to heed the "call of nature"; when this happens, the sensation of having to pass stools disappears for a while. The result is that waste products of digestion continue to accumulate in the rectum (the lower end of the large intestine), where they become large and hardened and increasingly difficult to pass.

Especially in older children and adolescents, chronic constipation is sometimes related to excessive worry, anxiety, fear, or other forms of emotional tension.

Frequent use of laxatives as well as certain drugs, such as intestinal antispasmodics, that inhibit normal motion of the bowels can also cause constipation.

Some cases of constipation are due to lack of fluid intake, since fluids help keep the stools soft.

Harsh laxatives should not be given to children. Indeed, any laxative should be given only with considerable caution. Be sure to follow label instructions for children's doses, and be sure never to exceed that dosage or extend the time limits that are noted. Mineral oil is a fairly safe means of softening the stools in children who are constipated; it also helps reduce straining during bowel movements. For children from about two to five years of age, the usual dosage is one tablespoonful in the morning and at night. This may be continued until loose or normal bowel movements occur on a daily basis. Commercial stool softeners can also be used to keep the bowel movements at a proper consistency, and infants can usually obtain prompt relief when their rectums are stimulated by a glycerin suppository.

If improvement is not noted within three days, or if a child suffers over a prolonged period from repeated bouts of constipation, parents should consult a doctor. Should ABDOMINAL PAIN be one of the symptoms of constipation, the child should also be taken to a doctor or other health-care professional (not necessarily an urgent situation) in case there is a more complex problem that requires prompt diagnosis and treatment.

Finally, parents should understand that for some children, just as in adults, having bowel movements only about three or four times a week is a normal pattern. So in many ways it is the degree of change from children's usual elimination pattern that signals constipation or diarrhea.

Crying

As parents well know, crying can indicate pain, fear, frustration, or a physical need. The subject is mentioned here mainly because of the tendency adults have of constantly telling a child *not* to cry.

An infant cries for a very basic reason: He or she has no other method of complaining verbally. Within the child's first weeks of life, parents usually learn to differentiate the pitch and volume used when infants are hungry, uncomfortable, afraid, tired, and so on.

As the child learns to talk, crying is still used as an emotional release. Even adults say, "I felt better after I had a good cry." Rather than eliminating the crying, parents should try to find out what is causing the child to cry. Often simple reassurance is all that is needed.

Cuts

Lacerations — small cuts of the child's skin — need little attention other than the following:

• Exert pressure to stop the bleeding
• Clean the wound with soap and water (parents may also use some mild antiseptic solution)
• Apply a nonstick dressing

Small cuts heal with little, if any, scarring.

If the edges of the wound are widely separated, use bandage strips to draw them together. If that does not work, suturing (stitching) by a physician may be required.

The wound should be observed for spreading redness or any drainage of pus, which might indicate an infection that requires medical attention.

Parents should keep a record of their children's immunization against TETANUS. For a clean, uncontaminated wound, a tetanus booster within the last ten years should suffice. For a dirty wound — for example, when there has been exposure to contaminated materials — the child should have had a tetanus booster shot within the last five years. If there is any doubt, consult the child's doctor or health-care professional.

Larger wounds, especially on the face, may leave prominent scars. It may take two years before facial scars disappear. Careful suturing by a qualified surgeon may minimize or even eliminate such scars.

D

Dandruff

The yellowish, greasy flakes that show up in the hair and on the shoulders and clothing of most Americans is the result of an inflammation of the scalp. The reason for the inflamed condition is unknown, but it occurs when the scalp becomes oily due to the sebaceous glands working overtime. However, dandruff (known technically as *seborrheic dermatitis*) may occur under exactly opposite conditions — when the hair and scalp are excessively dry.

Seborrheic dermatitis itself is not a serious condition; it is merely that the flakes are a source of self-consciousness and real or imagined social embarrassment. It is not curable, but it is controllable with special shampoos containing dandruff-fighting chemicals. It is also important to keep combs and brushes cleaned.

The only other problems with dandruff are that it can spread from the scalp beneath the hair to other parts of the head and neck and even other parts of the body; that a child with dandruff may have a greater chance of also having ACNE; and that dandruff sufferers tend to be more sensitive to chemicals than others.

Day Care and Illness

In this day and age of the two-career family, it is ever more common for parents to send their children to day care or early preschool. Depending on which side of the debate you are on — or, because of necessity, which side you have to be on — you either feel that the day-care situation does a fine job of socializing and preparing a child for future stages of life, or you believe that it is an unnatural warehousing for children who should be raised at home.

Whatever your personal view, one thing is clear: A day-care center is a key place for the spread of illness among children. Not that the centers themselves are dangerous, or breeding grounds, but because infants and toddlers, with immature and vulnerable immune systems, are exposed to other children who might have contagious or communicable illnesses such as flu, colds, infections, and so on. Normally, these sick youngsters would be kept at home until they got better, but without a parent at home to tend to them, they are often sent knowingly ill to day care, where they infect the others. Additionally, only licensed day-care centers require or recommend that the children they care for be immunized; those facilities with no such requirement lead to youngsters getting preventable diseases from one another.

There is really nothing that can be done about the situation. One cannot force parents of sick children to take a day or two off from work to tend their child. Neither should sick youngsters be forcibly isolated if they are feeling well enough to be up and about. And, for the most part, these are not serious illnesses that are caught at preschool settings; some may be annoying, some painful (such as ear infections), some long term (because the child continues to be reinfected with every visit to the center). In fact, some research indicates that although toddlers are very much affected and infected, after the age of three the number of illnesses tends to level off and even go down, because immunity has been built up early. This might mean fewer illnesses later during the school years.

It is important for parents to know that the likelihood of their child falling prey to childhood illnesses is high at any time, but almost certainly higher in a day-care setting.

Death of Parent or Sibling

As is true of many aspects of children's behavior, reactions to traumatic events will be modeled on what surrounding adults do. In the tragic event of a parent's or sibling's death, the survivors might best serve themselves and the child by *not* keeping a stiff upper lip. If the child is allowed to grieve openly and discuss feelings of loss, he or she may avoid or at least minimize the psychological problems that loss can cause. It is especially important that children be helped to understand that no matter what their secret moments of hate or wishing that the person would go away, they are not guilty of killing their mother, father, sister, or brother.

On the other hand, the child should not be given special privileges, in the sense of permitting behavior that was not previously acceptable or the formation of artificially close bonds, in vain efforts to make up for the loss. If symptoms of DEPRESSION develop, it may be helpful to enlist a professional who can assist the child in putting the death into a more appropriate perspective.

Destructive Behavior

This is a type of AGGRESSIVE BEHAVIOR, but rather than directing anger toward other people (including playmates) or himself or herself, the child attacks inanimate objects such as toys. It should be distinguished from activities in which children do, quite normally, take things apart out of sheer curiosity. However, the behavior should be observed carefully for frequency and intensity, for often it is what psychologists and psychiatrists call *displacement.* That is, the child may well wish to destroy a playmate, sibling, or parent but displaces the anger onto inanimate objects. If destructiveness is the rule rather than the exception, parents may wish to seek professional assistance.

Diarrhea

A condition in which the BOWEL MOVEMENTS are abnormally frequent (more than six in twenty-four hours) and consist of loose and watery stools. The diagnosis also applies to less frequent stools that are "explosive" and unusually voluminous. Diarrhea occurs fairly frequently in babies and very young children, especially in its milder forms. Causes include overfeeding; eating foods, including milk, to which the child is especially sensitive; or a digestive-tract infection. Especially in babies, diarrhea may accompany some other feverish illness, a sore throat, or an ear infection. Older children and adolescents may sometimes suffer from diarrhea caused by nervous excitement before examinations in school or social events.

In its more severe form, childhood diarrhea may feature stools mixed with slight traces of blood or pus. When this happens the child's doctor must be consulted immediately so that the cause can be determined and appropriate treatment begun. Serious diarrhea in infants is especially dangerous because of the possibility of DEHYDRATION.

Parents should become concerned if the number of stools exceeds six or eight, especially if vomiting is present. Changes in activity, dry lips and mouth, and decreased frequency of urination are also signs that the infant or child may be developing problems.

See also AMEBIC DYSENTERY, BACILLARY DYSENTERY, COLITIS, DEHY-
DRATION

Compare CONSTIPATION

Diet

For the first six to eight months of life, milk is the infant's main food.
Special formulas should be used if mothers cannot or do not wish to
breast-feed.

New mothers can obtain useful information from their child's
health-care professional about the best times and ways to add solid
foods to the baby's diet. Children differ, and there is no set rule about
what foods need to be added and when.

It is generally agreed that the child's own appetite will gradually
lead to seeking a balanced diet, especially when a variety of nutritious
and wholesome choices is offered. If a new taste is refused, do not force
the child to eat the food. Wait until he or she is a little older before
reintroducing the taste. Babies differ in their acceptance of new flavors and textures, and in Western culture almost all youngsters initially dislike highly spiced foods or unusually strong flavors.

In order to build a strong and healthy body, the child needs adequate amounts of carbohydrates, protein, fats, minerals, and vitamins. Precisely how much is difficult to say. Often it is a matter of
common sense: If the young child is thriving, attaining normal rates
of growth, and appears strong and healthy, he or she is probably
getting a diet that is adequate in essential nutrients.

There is some controversy concerning vitamins; some doctors recommend vitamin supplements until a child is about two years old,
after which time it is assumed that a well-balanced diet provides
ample amounts. Other practitioners disagree, believing that because
of extensive processing, foods that Americans eat rarely provide opti-
mal amounts of vitamins and minerals.

Another problem may arise with the common use of preservatives
in commercial foods. Some of these chemical additives have been tied
to the development of serious diseases, so, on the whole, parents are
best serving their children's needs when they serve fresh foods or ones
that are not packaged with chemicals intended to keep them from
spoiling.

Children's stomachs are small. They should not be expected to
consume huge quantities of food; in fact, they should be discouraged

from doing so because of digestive difficulties that may ensue. It is because of their small stomachs that children often prefer snacking to formal meals. Snacking is entirely appropriate, provided junk foods are avoided and the snacking is not done too close to mealtime.

Meals should be shared with the rest of the family. The child learns good table manners and gradually comes to enjoy mealtime conversations and the unhurried, peaceful atmosphere of sitting down to a good dinner. It is definitely not a time for arguing, coaxing, or forcing children to eat. Meals should be pleasant occasions; if they are presented that way, they will gradually discourage older children from overindulging in between-meal snacks as they grow to regard dinner as something to look forward to.

Nutritional problems in school-age children often come from skipping breakfast and eating unnutritious lunches. The latter may be a particular problem for children whose schools do not provide supervised lunches and who may spend lunch money on sweets or junk food. In adolescents, the opposite problem may occur. Suddenly concerned with their appearance and their attractiveness to members of the opposite sex, both girls and boys may put themselves on fad or crash diets that make exaggerated weight-loss claims. Parents should express sympathetic concern and reassure their child that the chunkiness somewhat common to the early teenage years will disappear as the young person grows and altered metabolism catches up with itself. Of course, when an adolescent is truly obese, parents should consider a medical consultation and the possibility of the child's undertaking a supervised program such as some of the professionally run summer camps devoted to weight loss.

About sweets: Again, common sense is the key. Prohibiting a toddler, child, or adolescent any sweets will be regarded for what it is: cruel and unusual punishment. On the other hand, overindulgence in candies, sundae toppings, and other sugary treats can lead to bad teeth and nutritional imbalances. One method of discouraging the overindulgence of sweets is to see that healthy snack foods such as carrots, celery, apples, and cheese are commonly munched on at home. If parents sit around devouring boxes of chocolate, the child can hardly be expected to develop a preference for health-promoting snack foods.

Finally, there is a direct connection between diet and behavior. Crankiness, irritability, lethargy, uncooperativeness, and many other unproductive behaviors can be influenced by improper diet. ATTENTION-DEFICIT DISORDERS have been linked to diet. Just as emotional problems can influence physical problems, bodily deficiencies can affect how the mind functions and how the child behaves. A practitioner's sensitivity to dietary factors may solve behavioral problems before the child is needlessly taken to a psychologist or psychiatrist.

See VEGETARIANISM

Dieting

In children a leveling off of an excessive gain pattern is what is needed, *not* weight loss. If the child is overweight, it is reasonable to limit excess sweets and starchy foods. Adequate amounts of protein, fats, and carbohydrates are needed, however, to ensure growth.

Adolescents' self-induced dieting should be strongly discouraged. This is particularly true in teenage girls whose marked weight loss may be connected to ANOREXIA NERVOSA, a serious condition that requires medical and psychiatric care.

Disobedience

The definition depends on what parents mean by "obedience." Parents need to discuss this matter between themselves and come to a common understanding of what they mean. This can help to ensure consistency in parental response to behavior that is considered unacceptable. Basically what concerned parents should seek is behavior that meets norms established for the child's age; a gradual socialization through which the child learns the give-and-take of everyday life; and the youngster's growing acceptance of standards of behavior that are acceptable within the home, at school, with other children, and in society at large.

In their zeal to be good parents, many people become overly controlling and too directive. Do not try to mold the child. Let the child make some mistakes and learn from the consequences. Provide general guidance and the means and support so self-respect is acquired. Do not control for the sake of control itself, and do allow the child some time alone, an interval when there are no orders or prohibitions. Having the parents' trust encourages the child to assume responsibility for his or her own behavior.

Before judging the child's behavior as disobedient, remember that from the very beginning, youngsters are striving for independence and self-expression. The way this is expressed often reflects the child's age. Infants tend to express frustration by crying. Toddlers, exploring new ways of getting around and of using newly discovered muscular powers and vocalizations, may throw a TEMPER TANTRUM if they do not get their own way. School-age children may pout, withdraw, or threaten extreme actions such as running away from home. As part of the power struggle between parent and child, conversations may be interrupted, chores left undone, or some behavior embarrassing to the parents be done in public. Adolescence, with its rebelliousness and its demands for real independence and self-assertion, can be a particularly trying time for parents, as it is for adolescents.

When parents view their child's behavior as continually disobedient, a critical self-appraisal of their parenting techniques may be helpful:

- Are both parents in agreement about expectations?
- Is there a consistency of response to unacceptable behavior?
- Is the child aware of the consequences of misbehavior?
- Are the methods of discipline fair, and does the punishment fit the crime?
- If threats of disciplining are made, are they consistently carried out?
- Is the child being unfairly used to vent parental anxiety or unrest?
- Is the child experiencing stress that has not been explored — perhaps trouble at school or problems with peers?
- Has good behavior been consistently rewarded, and is the child frequently reassured about love and acceptance?

If behavioral difficulties persist after all the above factors are inspected and legitimate attempts at change have failed, a discussion with the child's physician or health-care professional may be in order. Sometimes an objective view can help pinpoint the origin of a particular conflict.

Double Vision

Known technically as *diplopia*, double vision occurs when one object is seen as two objects. The condition may be present from birth, in which case the child usually learns to suppress the vision in one eye. It may be connected to a muscular imbalance called STRABISMUS (a squint). If this situation goes undetected and the child continues to suppress vision in one eye, one-eye blindness may result. But if the condition is diagnosed early — when the child is no older than five or six — it can be treated successfully so that the blindness does not become permanent. On rare occasions, double vision may be one of the first symptoms of BOTULISM, a severe form of FOOD POISONING caused by *Clostridium botulinum*, an organism that sometimes contaminates improperly preserved food. If botulism is suspected, prompt medical attention is mandatory, as the toxin (poison) affects the central nervous system and can cause paralysis of the heart and respiratory system. Double vision following a head injury is an ominous sign, and prompt medical attention is mandatory.

If parents notice any double-vision difficulties, they should take the child to an eye specialist at once. On the other hand, children often become quite adept, almost on an unconscious level, at concealing such problems, so a thorough eye examination at around age five is a wise move in any event.

Drowsiness, Unusual

The most common reason any child becomes drowsy is obvious — not enough sleep. Sleep patterns vary: Some infants sleep through the night by the time they are only 2 months old; others take a night feeding until they are 6 months or older. Babies may nap for up to 4 hours a day, so that they are sleeping about 12 to 14 hours out of every 24. Toddlers and young children often nap for 1 to 2 hours during the day and sleep about 8 to 10 hours during the night. Growing children and adolescents require at least 8 to 10 hours of sleep, sometimes more. Parents need to know their own children's patterns if they are going to judge what unusual drowsiness is.

Lack of sleep may occur for several reasons:

- The child goes to bed at an appropriate hour, but sleep does not come until sometime afterward
- The night may have been one of fitful, irregular sleeping
- The child may be worried about something and be afraid to go to sleep (a situation that may be worked out through a reassuring discussion, or may need professional help)

Children who are becoming ill may be unusually tired for a day or two before they develop other symptoms. Certain medications, especially antihistamines, cause drowsiness; so can DEPRESSION or emotional stress. ANEMIA may also produce an undue amount of FATIGABILITY, increasing the need for sleep.

Drug Usage

See ADDICTION, WARNING SIGNS OF

Dyslexia

There seems to be no single cause of dyslexia, which is a significant impairment in the development of reading skills. Many factors may be involved. Family histories suggest there may be some genetic component. A previous brain injury or infection could also contribute. The child, more often a boy than a girl, may also have shown slow motor development — that is, poor muscular coordination compared with age peers — and delayed language skills — that is, not talking as well as age peers. These are signs that parents can recognize while the child is still a preschooler.

It is of utmost importance for parents and teachers to understand that this impairment has nothing to do with the child's intellectual capacity. Indeed, many dyslexic children are as bright as nondyslexic children. They may, for example, have visual problems in which letters get fused or switched. Sounds may be confused, or the child may have trouble retaining what has gone before other letters or sounds. Both testing and training must be done by experts in the field, not by the average physician or the average teacher. Even after extensive correctional work, dyslexic children often continue to have some difficulties in spelling, reading, and comprehension throughout life. But with proper training, they can be taught to achieve levels that permit normal achievement in school. Training also greatly enhances their social acceptance.

For more information about dyslexia, call Orton Dyslexia Society, 800-ABCD-123, Monday through Friday, 9 A.M. to 5 P.M. eastern time.

E

Earache

Children's brief episodes of earache often reflect nothing more than pressure changes behind the eardrum; they are of no real significance and usually go away without any treatment. However, ear discomfort may occur because of:

- Infections
- The presence of a foreign object in the ear canal, such as insects or pea-size items such as stones or parts of toys
- Direct injury by poking a sharp object into the outer ear canal
- Enduring loud blasts

Sometimes pain may spread from the teeth or throat, and, in rare instances, otalgia (ear pain) can be caused by an inflammation of the nerve to the ear.

Infants or toddlers who cannot complain verbally may express ear discomfort by pulling at the ear, rubbing the side of the head, or even banging the head.

Frequent or persistent complaints warrant medical evaluation, especially if there is high fever or vomiting.

See EAR INFECTIONS

Emotional Withdrawal

This form of behavior — in which children or adolescents stop engaging in activities or relationships that previously seemed quite meaningful to them — may be a prominent feature of a childhood DEPRESSION, and if a clear pattern emerges of shunning friends and avoiding family and other social interactions, parents may want to seek professional help. Sometimes short-term family therapy is effective.

212

On the other hand, changing interests are a normal part of growing up. A youngster who last year seemed to do nothing but climb trees may suddenly opt for the studious and rather solitary activity of stamp collecting. Preadolescents and adolescents may go through painful periods of shyness as they try to cope with a new body image and newly awakened interests. Often children welcome discussions with their parents if they are approached in a serious, sympathetic, and nonteasing manner. If the areas of concern cannot be defined or if the withdrawal seems unduly severe and prolonged, check with the child's doctor. Perhaps counseling is in order, or perhaps there is some physical cause for the child's subdued state.

Eye, Foreign Body in

Flecks of foreign material, such as dirt or dust, are usually washed away by an immediate flow of tears. If this does not work, and gentle flooding with water or a sterile solution fails to dislodge the material, removal should be undertaken only by a doctor, nurse, or other practitioner who is trained to do so.

Larger objects, or ones that strike the eye with force, may scratch the cornea (the transparent covering in front of the eyeball) or the conjunctiva (the membrane that lines the eyelid and covers the white of the eye). The child is usually in extreme discomfort; tearing is common, and the eye looks quite red. Because tiny scratches in these delicate linings may provide an entry for harmful microorganisms, the child should be examined by a doctor. A special staining technique permits accurate location of the injury, and appropriate medications can be prescribed.

Any injury that penetrates into the eyeball is very serious. Never attempt to remove the object. Simply cover the eye with a cool wet cloth and rush the child to a doctor or the nearest emergency medical facility.

F

Fainting

A simple fainting spell — technically known as *syncope* — is not uncommon in childhood. It occurs because of a rapid drop in blood pressure in vessels supplying the brain and heart. It can, for example, be brought about by rising too quickly to an upright position. But children often faint when they are suddenly frightened, embarrassed, or in pain. Some children briefly lose consciousness over the simple removal of a splinter in the finger. Others, particularly older children or adolescents, may faint in response to some emotional strain that is experienced as overwhelming, such as having to give a speech or perform at a concert, or feeling clumsy when encountering someone who awes them.

The child may at first feel lightheaded and dizzy, and the skin becomes clammy. Occasionally there may be a brief twitching of muscles in the arms and face. Vision usually grows dim and fuzzy until the child simply blacks out and collapses, or gradually sinks to the floor or ground.

When the child complains of feeling faint, tilting the head downward at a 45-degree angle often helps prevent a total faint. Otherwise, simply help the child lie down if he or she has not already collapsed. Usually these attacks are brief and leave no ill effects afterward. Parents may wish to discuss their children's fainting spell(s) with a doctor, just in case some other condition such as abnormal heart rhythms or some SEIZURE DISORDER may be present. Syncope associated with strenuous activity (as in athletics) may be a symptom of a very serious cardiac (heart) abnormality, and a full medical evaluation is necessary.

Falling

Young children's behavior tends to be impulsive; they do not think before acting. As part of this pattern, children run or climb before they

214

look at what might be in their way. Frequent falls and bruises are the rule rather than the exception.

It is not possible for parents to protect youngsters from their own tangled feet. Nor should this necessarily be attempted; children need to test newly discovered muscular coordination. Falls and scraped legs are a normal part of young children's everyday lives.

Parents need, however, to be alert to signs of staggering or undue unsteadiness that might indicate an inflammation of the inner ear, where balance mechanisms are located. Other signs such as tremors, muscle weakness, and a wobbly gait might suggest a neurological disorder, as might the child's sudden fall to one side or the other even though he or she is not particularly active at the moment. These situations call for diagnosis and treatment by a doctor or health-care professional.

Fatigability

Along with the emotional mood swings seen in adolescence, there is an associated shift in energy levels. Many teenagers seem to require great amounts of sleep and may act as though they are always tired. Rapid growth, changes in metabolism, and the energy expended on emotional development are draining.

All children, including toddlers and youngsters, may become fatigued simply by too much physical exertion and insufficient rest or sleep. However, stress may add to children's fatigability. If gentle discussion cannot uncover family, peer, or school difficulties that may be stressful, some professional counseling may help. Parents should also keep in mind that unusual fatigability may indicate the subtle presence of some medical condition; therefore, a physical checkup might be in order.

See also DEPRESSION; DROWSINESS, UNUSUAL

Fears

Mental-health professionals often make a distinction between fear and anxiety. Fear is generally characterized as a reasonable reaction to something real that is generally looked upon as threatening or frightening. One could call a phobia unreasonable fear because it is highly exaggerated over what most people, including children, commonly experience. Anxiety is often tied to more vague fears that do not seem to be related to things that are readily seen, felt, or understood.

For most parents, the distinction may be more confusing than helpful. This is certainly true for the children themselves. Many fears are symbolic in origin and represent other anxieties, for example, dreading parental punishment or loss of parental love. Sometimes children become somewhat preoccupied with such concerns and behave anxiously in an overall way; that is, they may become jumpy, withdrawn, tearful, overexcited, or hard to get along with. If this becomes a marked problem, parents may want to discuss the matter with the child's doctor, who can help provide some guidance or perhaps make a referral for counseling.

In the vast majority of cases, the child's fears dissipate with calm parental reassurance and the child's own emotional growth as he or she gains more confidence.

Children should never be forcefully made to experience something they fear just to prove nothing will happen. For example, making a screaming child sit in a swing while you push it or shutting off the lights when the youngster is afraid of the dark only reinforces the fear. Children are apt to become even more fearful because parents have exposed them to a danger they consider very real, even if it is not. If the child is afraid of the dark, allowing a night-light in his or her room, coupled with gentle reminders that ghosts and monsters do not exist, is far more effective.

Obviously, everyone has fears. It is only when they seem to interfere with the child's functional level that any attention should be directed at correction. A direct behavioral approach seems to work better than endless discussions of the fear. In fact, this could backfire by turning the fear into an attention-seeking device.

Fecal Soiling

Children who begin to have accidents with bowel movements long after they are toilet trained may be doing so because they are trying to avoid having a bowel movement altogether.

This condition is seen more frequently in boys than in girls. The child may fight the urge to go to the bathroom to avoid interrupting play or other activities. Resistance during school hours may indicate the child is uncomfortable in a strange bathroom or is embarrassed by the need to go to the bathroom at all. In some cases, either a series of diarrheal episodes or having previously had a large and painful bowel movement may cause the child to be fearful that it will hurt again. Some authorities consider fecal soiling a sign of severe psychological disturbance, but, unless it is accompanied by other emotional symptoms, the situation does not require any special counseling. Whatever the cause, and often it simply cannot be determined, the child begins to resist going to the bathroom.

An early sign is cramping abdominal pain, which occurs because the child is holding back and fighting the urge to go. When successful, a day or two might pass without a bowel movement. When the child does go, the stool is large and likely to cause discomfort in passing.

Gradually, the period between bowel movements lengthens. Large amounts of stool are present in the lower intestine, so that underclothing may be soiled several times a day as fluid or small amounts of formed fecal material leak around the impacted stool. If this pattern persists longer than 6 to 12 months, the intestinal wall loses some of its normal tone because it is stretched by the frequent collection of waste matter. At this point, a physical cause for constipation and infrequent stooling exists.

What is necessary is to reestablish a normal bowel pattern and keep the bowel as free as possible from large collections of stool. This retraining should begin as soon as parents become aware of the problem, at which point they should consult the child's doctor. The physician may recommend enemas, stool softeners, or suppositories for rectal stimulation. This should be scheduled for the same time each day, whenever it is convenient. Harsh laxatives should not be used. As the child becomes accustomed to regular bowel movements and understands that he or she will have to go in spite of any holding, normal toilet habits are gradually relearned. Soiling is reduced because there is no excess buildup of stool, so corresponding embarrassment over accidents dissipates.

See also BOWEL MOVEMENT, ABNORMAL

Feeding Pattern Changes

The frequency and amount of feedings during infancy depend mostly on the baby's growth requirements. For the first few weeks, an infant wants to eat small amounts frequently. If too much is offered and taken, it will be graciously returned on the burping cloth or your shoulder.

After about six weeks, a feeding in the middle of the night is really not necessary. Substituting water helps. It may take a few days, but most babies will decide it is really not worth getting up at two o'clock in the morning for a couple of ounces of water.

Solid foods need not be introduced until an infant is about four months old, when, as a rule, the swallowing mechanisms and digestive system are better prepared to accept them. As more solids are introduced, the amount of milk needed diminishes. Since vegetables, fruits, and meats have fewer calories per ounce than milk, excessive weight gain is avoided. By the age of six or seven months, the infant should be on a schedule that approaches what childhood patterns will be:

• A carbohydrate source for breakfast: cereal and fruit
• Something filling but not fattening for lunch: vegetable and perhaps fruit
• A protein source for dinner: meat, vegetable

Amounts and consistency depend on what the baby can handle without choking or gagging. Finger foods, more to be played with than eaten, help develop coordination and allow the baby to begin to learn self-feeding.

When an infant reaches one year of age and weighs about 20 pounds, a rather dramatic decrease in appetite occurs. This often concerns parents, but it need not. The change merely means that the child has reached a predictable and normal slowdown in growth rate.

Compare APPETITE, CHANGES IN

Fever

A child is considered to have a fever when the body temperature, taken rectally, is above 100° (37.8° C). If the child's temperature cannot be taken rectally, you can gain some approximation by taking it orally or in the armpit (axillary region).

Accuracy of temperature may vary for many reasons other than body site, measuring technique, or presence of illness. Temperature of the surrounding air can cause some variation in body temperature. Vigorous play or environmental heat may cause readings of up to 100.5° F (38.1° C). Body temperature tends to swing from one time of day to another. This change, caused by varying secretions of cortisone by the adrenal glands, may cause lower readings in the morning and higher readings later in the day. If a child has been drinking cold liquids immediately before an oral temperature is taken, the reading will be artificially lowered.

A fever serves two purposes: alerting one to the possibility of disease and fighting, in a natural way, that disease or illness. In other words, vigorous attempts at fever reduction may sometimes delay accurate diagnosis and the body's own attempt to rid itself of sickness. *Therefore, except in young infants in the first few months of life, temperatures up to 102° F (38.9° C) need not be treated.*

Actually it is only in rare circumstances that a fever produces ill effects on the body. Temperatures below 107° F (41.5° C) do not cause brain damage; some infants and children have suffered no permanent injury as the result of short-term temperatures above 109° F (42.8° C). Parents often have an unreasonable fear that if children's fevers get too high, the youngsters will suffer a convulsion (see FEVER CONVULSION). As a matter of fact, if a seizure does occur, it often happens as the fever is just beginning its climb upward, not when it peaks. There is also a great deal of individual variation in sensitivity to temperature changes. Above all, since fever convulsions are not particularly dangerous, a concentrated attempt at keeping the child's temperature down serves little purpose.

Other factors, such as age and the presence of other signs or symptoms, are more important. For example, if a rectal temperature higher than 100° F (37.8° C) or lower than 98° F (36.6° C) occurs in an infant six weeks old or younger, that baby should be immediately taken for a medical examination. In very young babies, serious infections may be heralded by sudden fever or an abnormally low temperature.

The presence of signs and symptoms other than fever must be considered. For example, a temperature of only 102° F (39° C) in a child who has a stiff neck and is vomiting is far more serious than one of 104° F (40° C) in a youngster who looks well and is acting fairly well. In the first instance, the child may have MENINGITIS; in the second ROSEOLA, a rather harmless illness.

How does the child look and act as the temperature comes down? If activity and appearance improve, the illness is probably not urgent. But when children look as ill with 100.5° F (38° C) as they did at 103° F (39.5° C), parents should call a doctor at once.

What happens when the temperature increases rapidly? Parents frequently express concern about a temperature that suddenly shoots up to 105° F. Some fevers do progress rapidly, but no child's temperature is 98.6° F one minute and 105° F the next. It is simply that the parent did not know about it and was not measuring it when it was 101, 102, 103, and 104.

When the doctor agrees that it is best to try to bring the fever down, several things can be done. Aspirin or acetaminophen compounds can be administered, but parents should be sure to follow label directions very carefully. Aspirin should not be used if the child has an INFLUENZA-like illness or CHICKEN POX because of a possible link to a serious complication called REYE'S SYNDROME.

If the child's temperature is under 105° F, external cooling, such as by sponging, may not be necessary. However, it often offers the child some comfort and may help convince parents they are doing something for their sick child. Immersing a feverish child in cool water accomplishes little; nor does wrapping him or her in cold wet towels. The best method involves placing the naked child on a large towel. Using a washcloth or your hands, gently apply tepid water all over the body. Wait a few minutes for some drying to occur, then repeat the process. Check the child's temperature every 20 minutes. Do not be concerned if it has not come down; it may even go up a bit more. Sometimes it can be brought down in 20 minutes, sometimes it takes an hour.

Never use alcohol, alone or in water, for sponging. It may be absorbed into the body and cause toxic (poisoning) effects.

Parents can best be prepared to deal with children's fevers if they follow a plan. Early in the infant's life, discuss with the baby's doctor how he or she prefers to manage fevers, and when and under what circumstances the child's doctor should be called. Keep a fever-reducing medicine at home, in dosage forms appropriate for the youngster and approved by the doctor.

These steps should prepare you for most fever circumstances. However, when other symptoms are present along with the fever, or when a fever has persisted for more than 24 hours, call the child's doctor to discuss the condition.

See also TEMPERATURE in Appendix I: Norms and Values

Compare HYPOTHERMIA

Frustration

When needs or desires — even unrealistic ones — are not met, one feels a sense of anger and frustration. Part of a child's maturing concerns learning to live with frustration.

In their impulsiveness, infants and very young children seem to demand immediate gratification; they feel frustrated when their wants are thwarted. Parents should not strive to protect their children from all frustration. Youngsters constantly set up circumstances that test their newly discovered control of themselves and the environment. When they learn that no great ill befalls them if everything does not go exactly their way, they develop tolerance for disappointing events. They learn to deal with unsatisfied goals.

Learning adjustment and compromise is not easy. Children may react to seemingly trivial setbacks with anger, a crying spell, or refusal to continue an activity. Only if this pattern continues and seems to occur regularly might a parent consider seeking some professional help. A short ATTENTION SPAN, excess motor activity, ATTENTION-DEFICIT DISORDERS, and DEPRESSION may signal a disturbance beyond a young child's normal attempts at learning to deal effectively with frustration. As always, age is an important factor. A slip of a pencil may result in a crumpled drawing for a three-year-old. A slightly crooked wing may end up in a crushed airplane model for a six-year-old. If the child engaging in this intolerant behavior is, for example, eight or ten, then a professional consultation is probably in order.

Funerals

Before the age of seven or eight, the average child does not have much understanding of the finality of death. Even until age ten, children may be rather confused by the event.

Unless a youngster is unusually mature, viewing a body in a funeral home and witnessing all the grief surrounding a funeral may be extremely anxiety provoking. Children under age five or six should, if possible, be left at home if their parents must attend a funeral. Children who are seven or older may attend if they have been properly prepared. After age ten, children are less apt to have an adverse reaction, but even then some preparatory conversation is helpful.

Those who propose that even a very young child should attend funerals or viewings maintain that children need to learn to deal with loss and grieving. This may be true, but it is probably wiser to let them learn these things when they are older. The anxiety caused is likely to be far greater than any benefits. If someone close to the parents dies, children will learn something of grief by sharing their reactions.

Death should never be explained as sleep. Some children may try to avoid sleeping, for fear they might die. In families who believe in an afterlife, children can be told that the person who has died is now enjoying a different kind of existence in another place. If the concept of an afterlife is not part of the family's beliefs, the child can be told that the one who has died can no longer be part of their everyday lives, but that the survivors can take pleasure in remembering all the past experiences they have shared with the deceased.

If it is the child's own parent or sibling who has died, many other factors come into play; decisions must be individualized.

When there is really no way to avoid a child's attendance at a viewing or a funeral, or the family (and, on occasion, the child) feels strongly that participation is desirable, it is a good idea to see that the child is accompanied by someone who is not deeply involved in the grieving and who can offer some objective explanations of what is happening.

See also DEATH OF PARENT OR SIBLING

G

Gas, Unusual or Excessive

Infants are prone to excessive gas because, while taking milk, they tend to swallow air while vigorously sucking and gulping. If the air is not completely burped out, it forms bubbles that make their way through the digestive tract, causing cramping as they go.

For the infant who is having particular problems with gassiness, prevention can be achieved with frequent burping — after every ounce or two fed from a bottle, or every five to ten minutes during breast-feeding. Once the condition exists, you can try placing the baby on his or her abdomen on top of a heating pad or hot-water bottle — taking care to avoid burns. Stimulating the rectum with a lubricated thermometer or a glycerin suppository may facilitate passage of gas. A medication called simethicone is safe and can be given orally to help break up the gas bubbles.

As the child grows and the diet expands, foods high in nitrogen content may cause excessive gas. Cabbage and beans are notorious offenders. Some older children may develop the habit of swallowing air or may do so when they are anxious.

MILK ALLERGY or intolerance to lactose (milk sugar) may cause excess amounts of gas to be formed. MALABSORPTION SYNDROME can result in gassiness because food is inadequately digested. Cramping, bloody diarrhea, and excessive gassiness may be symptoms of other diseases; a medical evaluation is necessary to arrive at an accurate diagnosis and plan appropriate treatment.

See LACTASE DEFICIENCY/LACTOSE INTOLERANCE

Growth Failure

Some children may simply be shorter than others, particularly if their parents are not tall, since genetic influences play a major role in determining height. As long as children do not fall too far from their

223

established pattern, there is no cause for concern. A child's own individual previous growth rate is more valuable than statistical comparisons with other children of similar ages.

Infants grow very rapidly in their first year of life. In the first six months they generally double their birth weight, and in the next six months they triple it. At the end of the first year, they will have grown about ten inches. Afterward the pattern slows. Each year generally adds from three to seven pounds in weight and about two inches in height. During adolescence a growth spurt occurs, with as much as six to eight inches of added height.

If parents have maintained good records and note that a child has definitely slowed in his or her normal growth pattern, medical advice should be sought. A pituitary or some other hormonal imbalance may be at fault. Certain illnesses may interfere with growth, but when they are treated appropriately the child can catch up.

H

Hair, Loss and Thinning of

Hair growth occurs in cycles. During one of the cycles in this process, it is normal for the human scalp to lose from 50 to 100 hairs each day. Some of this loss may be noticed during combing or brushing, but usually it simply falls away unnoticed and is replaced by new hair. (Your child is not going bald.)

"Plucking" may contribute to hair loss. Some children — often those given to habits such as thumb sucking — may pull and pluck at the scalp until hair shafts are broken and a baldish spot appears. This is often done unconsciously; when the pulling stops, the hair grows back naturally. Similar bald spots may result from too much tension from barrettes or tight ponytails, or when infants lie on their backs for most of the day.

Certain fever-producing illnesses as well as emotional stress, injuries, and adolescents' crash diets may interrupt normal hair-growth cycles. But if the precipitating cause is not repeated, a full head of hair will return over a period of several weeks. (Actually only about one quarter of the total number of hairs fall out, but the loss can be quite noticeable.)

A condition thought to be related to the body's immune system may cause very sudden hair loss in well-outlined patches. Cortisone compounds can speed hair regrowth, but even though these medications can be obtained without a doctor's prescription, they should not be used until a physician or health-care professional diagnoses the problem and recommends such treatment.

Halitosis

See BAD BREATH

Head Banging

Impacting the head against any surface, such as when infants some-times rock against the crib mattress, apparently provides rhythmic relaxation as they are going to sleep. Except when an EAR INFECTION is present, head banging may be a child's attempt to relive the early security of the crib.

Children rarely persist in the behavior after they reach the age of four, although some continue it into the early school years. Providing an air of relaxation at bedtime may help. Under no circumstances should the child be physically restrained.

Head Injury

The heavy, bony casing of the skull is normally an efficient protector of the delicate brain inside it. Unless the skull is severely fractured, the bone acts as a barrier between penetrating wounds and soft nerve tissue. However, the skull cannot prevent the brain from being af-fected by a CONCUSSION when the head is jolted.

Any fairly serious blow to the head is an immediate alarm to call for medical help. If there is any likelihood of a fractured neck or spine, it is best to leave the child in the position in which he or she was found. If the victim is unconscious, protect the airway by keeping the head stable while thrusting the jaw forward and immediately clearing any fluid in the mouth before it obstructs breathing. Otherwise, try not to move the child until medical personnel arrive. If circumstances are such that the child must be moved, do so with extreme caution. Sometimes gently lifting the body onto a hard surface, such as a wooden plank, provides protection against further movement as the child is being transported to an emergency facility. Any slight bleeding from the ear or nose or bruising around the eye should be regarded as potentially serious signs.

A very severe blow that damages the skull may cause compression of the brain. Pieces of broken bone may press against the brain's surface. The general swelling that accompanies any fracture, which can show on the surface as a puffy area of scalp or skin, can also cause inside swelling that presses against brain tissue. Finally, any bleeding inside the skull will compress the jellylike brain within the hard, bony casing into which it fits so closely.

If the compression is severe enough, it can cause unconsciousness and even death. Unlike the instant knockout of a concussion, unconsciousness develops gradually in cases of compression. The child may pass through stages of headache, irritability, nausea and vomiting, and make uncontrolled jerky movements before becoming drowsy and losing consciousness. This may take minutes or hours, depending on how much and how fast the pressure is building.

Although any head injury, particularly if followed by a period of unconsciousness, must be considered a true medical emergency, parents should be relieved to know that children have a remarkable ability to recover from what seems to be, and often is, a very serious head injury.

For more information, the National Head Injury Foundation offers the following toll-free number: 800-444-NHIF.

Headache

Headaches are not uncommon in children. It is rare, however, that they signal any serious disease.

Nonetheless, it is helpful to a doctor, and ultimately to the child, if parents make notes about their child's complaints of headaches:

- Is the discomfort localized or diffuse?
- Is it one-sided?
- Where did it begin?
- Is there anything that seemed to bring it on?
- How long does it last?
- How often do they occur?
- At what time of the day does it tend to come on?
- Is there a family history of similar headaches?
- Are there any other signs or symptoms present, such as vomiting?

Migraine headaches may occur at any time during childhood or adolescence. A strong family background makes the diagnosis more likely. Migraines tend to occur suddenly and sometimes are preceded by the sensation of lights flashing or there being wavy lines in front of the eyes. The pain is severe and throbbing and is often confined to one side of the head. Nausea and vomiting are fairly common. Children affected just want to lie down in a dark room and be left alone, which is good therapy, since sleep often takes the headache away. A physician's evaluation is needed in order to determine the best course of drug treatment. Parents can help the child understand that he or she may have these headaches off and on throughout life, but that they are not serious.

Tension headaches are unusual in younger children and are more prevalent in adolescents. The pain arises from fatigue and/or stress, usually starting in the muscles in the back of the neck, then proceeding upward along each side of the forehead. The pain is dull and aching, and may worsen as the day progresses. There is no vomiting or other symptoms except perhaps for irritability. Aspirin generally offers relief, and sleep seems to clear the headache altogether.

Along with muscle aching, a headache may be an early feature of INFLUENZA or other VIRAL INFECTIONS. But contrary to popular opinion, eyestrain and a need for corrective lenses are not associated with headaches. Children with SINUSITIS or who are suffering from DEPRESSION or other emotional problems may also complain of headaches.

Because headaches are not an everyday occurrence in children, parents often tend to think the worst if their child gets them. The fear of brain tumor seems to be high on the list. However, this condition, although ranking high in incidence of childhood tumors, is really quite rare. Episodes of headache are caused by increased pressure within the skull. As the pressure increases, so does the incidence of vomiting, which may be projectile, that is, the material may shoot out in an arc. Obviously medical attention is necessary, but fortunately, very few parents ever encounter this situation.

Severe headaches may also accompany other medical conditions such as SEIZURE DISORDERS or the emergency illnesses MENINGITIS and ENCEPHALITIS. Both meningitis and encephalitis are associated with fever, vomiting, and a stiff neck, serious signs that alert parents to the need for quick medical attention.

For more information about headaches, their treatment, and physician referral, call the National Headache Foundation at 800-843-2256.

Hearing Loss

Parents can usually determine whether a child has a hearing problem by:

- Certain patterns of behavior (for example, the child's seeming to ignore noise or showing an unusually limited attention span)
- Difficulties a toddler encounters trying to speak
- Simple tests such as measuring the distance at which the child can hear a whisper or a watch ticking

Specialized testing is necessary to determine the extent of hearing loss and the range of frequencies that can be heard. One method of testing, called speech audiometry, uses a recording of spoken words played through headphones at varying degrees of loudness. This method has an advantage over the tone method because it permits the tester to determine more precisely if the hearing problem is caused by conductive DEAFNESS or nerve deafness. Speech audiometry also allows an assessment of the value a hearing aid might provide to the child.

In the United States, it is fairly standard practice to provide free hearing tests to children of school age, especially when they are in kindergarten or first grade. If a hearing problem is discovered, parents should immediately seek outside professional assistance for the child.

Deafness, if present, is a particularly serious problem in the child's development and education. Children need to be able to communicate their feelings and thoughts and to be able to share in the experiences of others. There are schools for the deaf that specialize in teaching language and lipreading, together with other methods of communication such as finger spelling and other forms of sign language.

It is generally accepted, however, that the successful development of skills in lipreading and speech is more important than sign language. Heavy dependence on sign language may lead the child to withdraw gradually from social involvement with those whose hearing is normal.

More information may be obtained by calling the following toll-free numbers: Better Hearing Institute, 800-424-8576 or 800-EAR-WELL, Monday through Friday, 9 A.M. to 5 P.M. eastern time (703-642-0580 in Virginia); Deafness Research Foundation, 800-535-3323; Hearing Aid Help Line, 800-521-5247, 9 A.M. to 5 P.M. eastern time; Hearing Screening Test (on-line hearing test), 800-222-EARS, Monday through Friday, 9 A.M. to 6 P.M. eastern time (800-345-3277 in Pennsylvania); National Association for Hearing and Speech, 800-638-8255 (301-897-8682 in Maryland); TRIPOD Grapevine, 800-352-8888, 8 A.M. to 6 P.M. Pacific time.

Heartbeat, Irregular

An abnormally fast heartbeat is called *tachycardia*. It may be associated with hyperthyroidism (an overactive thyroid gland) or some form of heart disease. In *paroxysmal tachycardia*, the heart suddenly starts to beat rapidly, a fluttering sensation is felt in the chest, and the child may feel faint. Often the episode ends abruptly after just a few minutes. These symptoms can occur in a child with a perfectly healthy heart, but a doctor should be consulted so that a proper diagnosis can be made and treatment can be provided to relieve the distress and anxiety these episodes cause. Sometimes medication is prescribed. Sometimes simple home remedies, such as sucking on crushed ice or lying flat on the floor, are recommended.

An abnormally slow heartbeat is called *bradycardia.* It may occur in a perfectly healthy child at times, especially in youngsters who are athletes. If not accompanied by faintness or dizziness, it is often considered a healthy sign in the sense of longevity and relative immunity to high blood pressure and other illnesses.

Arrhythmia is the name given to an abnormal rhythm or disturbance of the heartbeat. Some children have a harmless condition known as *sinus arrhythmia*, in which the pulse rate increases when they breathe in and decreases when they breathe out. It is rarely associated with any other symptoms or disease processes.

Hoarseness

During childhood the most common reason for hoarseness is an acute infection such as CROUP or LARYNGITIS. If they are associated with breathing difficulties, these illnesses require emergency medical care. When breathing is not affected, providing moisturized air with vaporizers or bathroom steam and plenty of fluids helps lessen symptoms.

Hoarseness may come from voice overuse. Children tend to be noisy; extended periods of loud play or screaming may cause them to become hoarse. Even with normal voice use, children may tire their vocal cords. Rest and quiet cures the problem.

Hoarseness that develops slowly and becomes progressively worse could indicate a papilloma (singer's nodes), small nonmalignant tumors that usually recede without surgical removal.

Occasionally newborn infants have a softening of the supporting structures around the vocal cords, or one cord may be paralyzed. Neither of these disorders causes any long-term problem, and the difficulty is usually outgrown.

Homosexuality

At least occasional homosexual behavior — an individual's preference for sexual contact and/or romantic involvement with members of the same sex — is seen in many species. Because preteens frequently form very close attachments with same-sex friends with whom they may engage in a little sexual exploration, authorities used to believe that most older children went through a homosexual stage that they outgrew.

However, this seems not always to be the case. Rarely does some crisis in gender identity play a role in a preference for homosexuality. These young people seem quite clear about their maleness or their femaleness, but for reasons that none of the multiple theories has ever conclusively proved, they simply find their affectional needs best fulfilled by persons of the same sex.

For most, the conflict does not surround their homosexuality; rather, it concerns familial and societal responses and worry about how disapproval and not fitting in may interfere with leading a normal and productive life.

Parents may feel angry, or feel they are at fault — as if homosexuality were something to fault or be blamed for. It is important that love prevail and parents not abandon their own child. Frank, open, supportive discussions are helpful to both the parents and the child. Consulting a physician or other professional should not be done as a means of altering the young person's thoughts and feelings, but only to make sure that he or she is comfortable in this choice and is fully aware of the implications of swimming against the mainstream.

In those instances in which the individual actually wishes to assume a heterosexual life-style, counseling can sometimes be helpful. But parents are cautioned not to be overly optimistic about change. In general, sheer acceptance even if parents do not actually understand goes a long way in strengthening family bonds and in helping the child achieve self-respect and balance. Some parents have found support groups such as Parents of Gays helpful.

Hyperactive Behavior

The term used to be used as a diagnostic category; now hyperactivity — behavior in which a child seems to be constantly moving, and in which a child's activity level is far greater than one would expect in children of that age — is considered to be part of an ATTENTION-DEFICIT DISORDER.

Children who are hyperactive are extremely loud and noisy. Crowded places stimulate increased levels of purposeless movement. Shopping and visiting become major undertakings, and baby-sitters may refuse to sit with a hyperactive child. Such children climb, run, fidget, and squirm. Teachers report disruptive behavior. Not even sleep is restful; in the morning, bedclothes may be on the floor in a tangled mess.

Understandably, but unfortunately, many hyperactive children are seen as simply misbehaving. They are yelled at and disciplined for something they cannot control, which increases the child's anger at what is perceived as unfair treatment.

The cycle must be broken if the child is to mature properly. But treatment should not be undertaken lightly. A thorough evaluation by a team of medical and psychological professionals is needed. Both medications and environmental changes may be recommended. A relationship to diet and the adverse effects of some food additives may also play a role. In any event, parents are urged to seek help, otherwise learning will be impossible and the child's chances for success as an adult will be severely hampered.

I

Imaginary Friends

Until they are around the age of four or sometimes older, children have a natural difficulty separating reality from imagination. Unless this confusion permeates most of the child's everyday life, or episodes of EMOTIONAL WITHDRAWAL are present, this rich imagination is actually a good thing. It permits a child to test newly learned social skills, communicate certain thoughts and feelings, and boost creative thinking. Even when a child has playmates and siblings, he or she may create a very special friend with whom special moments can be shared.

Parents should never scold or tease the child. At the same time, neither should they go overboard in integrating the imaginary friend into the entire family scene. As long as children understand that this is part of their own "pretend" world, they should be allowed to enjoy an imaginary friend without interference.

Immunization

In active immunization a vaccine is given that stimulates the body's protective mechanisms to prepare antibodies that fight the disease when it is encountered. Passive immunization is used when an individual has already been exposed to the disease.

It is now routine in the United States and Canada to immunize against MEASLES, MUMPS, RUBELLA (German measles), POLIOMYELITIS, Hemophilus influenza type B (Hib), and a triad called DPT: DIPHTHERIA, PERTUSSIS (whooping cough), and TETANUS (lockjaw). The following schedule of vaccination is currently recommended by the American Academy of Pediatrics:

- 2 months — DPT, OPV (oral polio virus vaccine), and Hib vaccine
- 4 months — DPT, OPV, and Hib vaccine
- 6 months — DPT and Hib vaccine

- 15 months — MMR (measles, mumps, rubella) and Hib vaccine
- 18 months — DPT, OPV, and Hib vaccine
- 4–6 years — DPT and OPV
- 10–12 years — MMR or measles vaccine alone
- 14–16 years — TD (tetanus and diphtheria toxoids)

Please note that it is currently recommended that infants receive an Hib vaccine at 2, 4, 6, 15 and 18 months of age. Immunization schedules differ for those children who are not immunized during their first year. Contact the child's physician for a revamped immunization schedule.

Immunization procedures have drastically reduced the deaths and complications from these once lethal diseases. Although some minimal risks are involved, no child should be denied this protection. Parents whose beliefs prohibit the unnecessary introduction of medical substances into children's bodies should give extremely careful consideration to the consequences of exposing nonimmunized children to the germs and viruses they are likely to encounter in everyday life. Of course, if the child has had an IMMUNIZATION REACTION, tends to be allergic, or is already sick, these situations must be discussed with the doctor whenever any immunization is planned.

Immunization Reaction

The vast majority of children experience little or no reaction to the routine series of immunizations. Practicing pediatricians strongly believe that the benefits of protection far outweigh the slight chance of hazard. However, because potentially serious complications can occasionally arise, parents should be aware of these risks. Also, if a child has had any adverse reaction to previous immunizations, the doctor should be told. These signs include:

- Convulsion
- Shock
- Fever over 105° F
- Screaming or crying for more than three hours. When this is a significant sign, the infant or toddler cannot be calmed no matter what is done.
- Lethargy or sleepiness for more than three hours. The child who falls asleep and is aroused only with great difficulty, even at feeding

time, may have a more serious reaction with the succeeding injection.

Clearly, a parent should call the doctor when any of these signs appear. Immunizations should not be given to a child who has an acute illness more serious than a cold, and disorders of the nervous system (such as a SEIZURE DISORDER) may rule against immunization.

The common childhood immunizations and their possible reactions are:

- *Oral polio vaccine.* No immediate side effect is seen. Only one in as many as ten million doses will be associated with development of the disease in the child or in some unimmunized person with whom he or she comes in contact. Permanent crippling or even death may occur. Anyone with an illness that impairs body defense mechanisms should not be given this vaccine.
- *DPT* (DIPHTHERIA, PERTUSSIS, TETANUS). Most children will have some soreness and even swelling at the injection site. Fevers may occur in the first 24 to 48 hours, with temperatures of 102° to 103° F. In about 1 out of every 7,000 doses given, somewhat more serious side effects may be seen: high fever (temperature over 103° F), convulsions, undue irritability, extreme lethargy, and shock (signaled by paleness, breathing difficulty, and unresponsiveness). Much more rarely, permanent brain damage may occur in 1 out of every 310,000 children immunized. On even rarer occasions, death is a possibility.
- *MMR* (MEASLES, MUMPS, RUBELLA). The MMR is one vaccine that immunizes against all three diseases. (Children can also receive a separate vaccine for each one.) About 20 percent of children immunized get a rash or fever ten days to two weeks after immunization. Usually the fever is low grade, but the temperature might reach 103° F. Although this has not been confirmed, it is said that ENCEPHALITIS (an inflammation of the brain) may occur in one out of every million children who get the measles vaccine; the incidence of encephalitis in an individual who contracts natural measles is one in a thousand.

A mild swelling of the salivary glands along the underside of the jaw may follow a mumps injection, but this clears spontaneously. The rubella vaccine may be followed by aching or swelling of the joints, which is usually noticed one to three weeks after the injection; the swelling clears in two or three days.

Although parents should be aware of these reactions and risks and should be sure to discuss with the physician any previous adverse reactions, they should be reassured that routine immunization has dramatically improved the health of children in the United States. For example, before the pertussis vaccine was used, about 265,000 cases of whooping cough occurred each year, with 7,000 deaths. By the early 1980s, there were only 1,000 to 3,000 cases with 5 to 20 deaths a year. The disease itself is extremely dangerous because it can cause long-term problems with the lungs or brain and may result in death.

Avoidance of immunization is not advised. A lengthy car trip carries a far greater chance of a bad outcome than all the immunizations combined. Yet for one reason or another, many parents are not taking their children to be immunized, or are not going through with the full scope of vaccinations, so the last few years have seen mini-epidemics of measles and pertussis. These are totally preventable diseases.

For those whose children have been injured in any way by immunization vaccines, the 1986 National Childhood Vaccine Injury Act helps to compensate victims through a trust fund set up from tax monies paid by pharmaceutical companies. Information can be obtained by contacting the National Vaccine Injury Compensation Program, Parklawn Building, Room 7-90, 5600 Fishers Lane, Rockville, MD 20857, or by phoning 301-443-6593.

Incest

Strictly speaking, sexual intercourse between two people closely related by blood is considered incest. Modern descriptions include not only intercourse but any degree of excitation by fondling, and the definition may also be expanded to include stepparents, grandparents, adult caretakers, or other relatives.

Over the past few years, there seems to have been a steady increase in media coverage of this serious problem. It remains somewhat unclear whether this reflects lowered barriers about reporting the violation and discussing the subject, or whether there is an actual increase in cases of incest.

Of reported incidents, about 95 percent involve girls between the ages of 2 and 18, most of whom have had their first such experience before the age of 12. Three quarters of the time the offender is either the father or stepfather, and most such involvements last for more than a year. Only 1 percent of incestuous relationships are initiated by adult females. Some authorities believe that sibling incest may be even higher than adult-child contact. It is probably reported less frequently, and, unless there is an extreme difference in age, it seems certain that the experience entails a great deal less trauma because it involves two children who probably engage in sex play by mutual consent, rather than an adult-child relationship in which the adult is *always* the responsible party. The myth about little girls being provocative should be relegated to the limbo it deserves. No matter what a young girl's behavior, it is the adult who bears responsibility for initiating sex play with a child.

It is not clearly understood why incest, usually occurring between father and daughter, occurs. The families tend to be private and without much outside social interaction. Mother-daughter roles may be reversed in the household. The fathers are often very strict and quite controlling of their daughters' lives. The father may have been exposed to incestuous relationships in his own childhood home. Many times the mothers are sexually remote and, knowingly or unknowingly, contribute to the affair by arranging to be away from home, leaving the father and daughter alone. There is typically little emotional interaction between the mother and the daughter, and the child is not given the strength and self-respect necessary to resist abnormal advances. Overall, there is a distortion of family dynamics that involves all family members. Secrecy becomes of vast importance.

A child or teenager who is being sexually abused may show signs of EMOTIONAL WITHDRAWAL or DEPRESSION. FEARS and phobias may become pronounced. NIGHTMARES, SLEEP PROBLEMS, and REGRESSIVE BEHAVIOR such as THUMB SUCKING may be clues. Vague ABDOMINAL PAIN and HEADACHES may signal the emotional stress being suffered.

If it is believed that a child is being molested, a report to a child-abuse agency or protective service is mandatory. What follows — agency intervention, possible severance proceedings, a court order to prevent visitation rights, and so on — may be uncomfortable for all concerned. However, without intervention the consequences are even worse, interfering with the child's normal development and most likely leading to very severe emotional problems that may, in turn, affect the victim's own relationships with future children.

The child or teenager should not be questioned about the specifics of the events any more than is necessary. Support and understanding are crucial, and the girl must be helped to comprehend that this is not her fault and that any future attempt should be reported immediately. Family therapy will most likely be required, and in many cases the child may be removed from the family, at least during a period in which the father is assigned to a counseling group that specializes in the problems of rape and incest.

Insomnia

See SLEEP PROBLEMS

J

Jaundice

This yellowish coloring of the skin and often of the whites of the eyes is caused when a bile pigment called bilirubin, a breakdown product of the oxygen-carrying part of red blood cells, gets deposited in skin tissues. Jaundice is not a disease but a symptom. Therefore, it is always a signal that medical evaluation is necessary.

Jaundice is present at birth or is observed during the first week of life in approximately 60 percent of full-term babies and about 80 percent of premature infants. This generally occurs because the bilirubin is not broken down, usually because of the immaturity of the liver or some congenital (present-at-birth) abnormality in the biliary tract. In most cases, the symptoms disappear spontaneously, although the nursing and medical staff will be alerted to any underlying disorder that should be investigated and treated. Whatever the causative problem — generally in the liver or gallbladder — treatment is necessary to prevent the child from developing a more serious condition.

See HEPATITIS

Jaw Pain and Swelling

Jaw pain and swelling are most frequently caused by a dental abscess. The infection may spread deeply into the bone if the situation is untreated.

SWOLLEN GLANDS may cause a great deal of discomfort, as does a FRACTURE of the jaw. Tumors and cysts of the jaw develop slowly, with swelling and pain being late symptoms.

Caffey's disease, marked by painful jaw swelling and a low-grade fever, may occur in infants. The cause of the disorder is unknown. Symptoms may be present for several months, but no treatment is effective. Eventually the swelling goes down and no deformity remains. If causes such as a cut or infected hair follicle are at fault, antibiotics will be needed to clear the infection.

L

Lactase Deficiency/Lactose Intolerance

This is a deficiency in the intestinal enzyme lactase, leading to inability to absorb lactose in milk, resulting in gassiness, bloating, diarrhea, and other abdominal discomfort.

This condition is considered hereditary, although it can suddenly surface as a side effect of a bout with a serious intestinal disease such as ulcerative COLITIS, viral GASTROENTERITIS, or tropical sprue. It tends to affect blacks and Asians far more than it does whites, and sufferers number in the millions.

Although not a serious condition, it is certainly a painful, embarrassing, and inconvenient one. In the United States, children's diets seem to revolve around milk. To be unable to drink it without getting pain or flatulence seems to be a cruel joke.

The problem is that the sugar in milk, called lactose, is normally broken down in the intestine by the enzyme lactase. It is then absorbed by the body. But when there is insufficient lactase to act on the lactose, the lactose is not absorbed; it is acted on by intestinal bacteria and begins to ferment, causing the familiar gas and bloating symptoms. It all goes back to nature, where most animals do not drink milk (that is, they no longer suckle) after their brief infancy, and so as their lactase naturally declines it causes no problem for them whatsoever. We humans, however, continue to drink milk, although our lactase dwindles (from about age three or four) as it does with our fellow mammals.

Despite its linkage with high cholesterol and allergies, milk is a staple in this country, and it is difficult for us to imagine a child being healthy without drinking it. There are, therefore, ways around the effects of lactase deficiency/lactose intolerance. First, it has been noticed that if sensitive children sip milk slowly instead of gulping it down, it gives the little remaining lactase in the intestine (it is rare for all of it to vanish) a chance to work to digest the small amounts of milk thrown its way. A few weeks on a soybean milk formula gives the intestine time to heal, and the problem should clear up. Children who continue to suffer discomfort or diarrhea after they have drunk milk should be given substitute products as recommended by a doctor or health-care professional. Some dairy products produce little or no deficiency symptoms; these include yogurt and buttermilk. In addition, there are products, such as Lactaid, available in groceries and supermarkets that, when added to milk, neutralize the lactose and make the liquid drinkable without problems; some companies also sell their own brand of milk with the delactosing already performed at the bottling plant.

The other response to lactase deficiency/lactose intolerance is to just go ahead and drink milk. The problems will remain, but they are more annoying than severe, and if the trade-off is worth it, then there is no reason that a choice to accept the consequences should not be made.

For more information about lactase deficiency/lactose intolerance, you may call the toll-free number of the company that makes Lactaid at 800-257-8650.

See MALABSORPTION SYNDROME, MILK ALLERGY

Learning Disabilities

Problems learning in school do not necessarily mean the student is not intelligent. Often, quite the contrary is the case. Some very bright pupils have trouble with schooling because of one or another obstacle in their capacity to process the information provided them. These obstacles may derive from any of a number of sources: Some may be genetic, while others may be learned or caused by the social atmosphere in which the child grows up. But a learning disability does not mean a child is unable to learn; it merely means that he or she has troubles doing the work within a certain system of teaching style. Given another form of instruction — say, verbal instead of written — the child might shine.

Some learning disabilities may be medically related — for example, allergies and ear infections could cause hearing problems that might stand in the way of a child's learning in a standard classroom setting — and, thus, a child should be examined at regular intervals, and more frequently if learning problems, sudden or otherwise, arise.

Some of the better known learning disabilities are:

- *Dyslexia*. This is a difficulty in comprehending written language, or to use language as a tool.
- *Dysnomia*. This is a difficulty in remembering and verbalizing words and the names for objects. This is one of a number of word-retrieval disabilities, and is sometimes called *aphasia*.
- *Concentration difficulties*. These may be medical in origin, or could be the signs of a gifted but bored child.

If your child seems to be exhibiting frustration with school, poor marks, poor or nonexistent writing skills or handwriting legibility, reluctance to do homework or to discuss the day's learning — and if you know that your child is bright and not otherwise a problem — you should discuss the situation with the school counselor. A physical examination may be in order, including a hearing test and an eye exam. And you may need to consult with a learning disabilities specialist who may want to test your child and suggest courses of therapy. This is a complex problem and needs to be treated early to avoid the unnecessary and uncalled for tracking of bright children into improper paths for them.

See also ATTENTION-DEFICIT DISORDERS

Leg Cramps

Children most often suffer leg cramps because of excessive running, climbing, and general horseplay. After a few minutes, the pain goes away, and they are off and running again.

Sometimes a day's activities will cause cramping later, so that the child awakens during the night, crying or complaining. A warm bath, a children's dose of an aspirinlike medication, and massaging the legs often relieve the pain. Symptoms may persist over several days or weeks, but the problem eventually goes away by itself as the child's leg muscles strengthen.

Leg cramping and other muscular cramps may plague teenage athletes at times of extreme exertion. Plenty of liquids should be taken to replace the loss of body fluids and the imbalance of salts that cause the discomfort.

On rare occasions, improper footwear may cause muscles to tire too quickly, so that a child or adolescent suffers leg pain or cramping.

Lice Infestation

Infestation with lice, a condition known as *pediculosis*, is far more common than the general public tends to think. Although it most often is a problem when a child's hair, skin, and clothing are not kept clean, children can and do inadvertently acquire lice by coming into contact with infested people or articles, for example, a comb, a hat, or someone else's jacket. Most schools report at least one outbreak of lice during each school term, so parents should not be ashamed or feel that their household is dirty if children become infested.

First signs are usually intense itching, irritation, and inflammation or redness of the skin. Lice are frequently found on the scalp and in the hair, but they can also be found on the body, especially on hairy parts. The eggs or nits have small grayish bodies and stick to the hair and cannot be brushed off; they take about two weeks to hatch. The eggs of body lice tend to be laid in clothing and underclothing, especially along seams. Body lice cause itching across the abdomen and back and sometimes produce hivelike rashes. Pubic lice affect not only the pubic area but also the thighs and lower abdomen.

Probably the first rule of treatment is to avoid scratching, which can cause a bacterial infection. The hair should be thoroughly lathered with a special shampoo, then rinsed and dried. Dip a fine-toothed comb into vinegar and run it through the hair repeatedly from the scalp outward. Nits can also be removed one by one with tweezers if parents are patient and take their time.

Although some lice medications are available without a prescription, it is best to ask the child's doctor or health-care professional for a recommendation. A cream or lotion containing 1 percent gamma benzene hydrochloride, available by prescription, is often effective when used as the doctor instructs. Treatment of lice on the eyelashes can be started by applying a Vaseline-like product to the eyelid margins, but only a physician should attempt removal.

If one child is infested, everyone in the family should be carefully inspected and treated if necessary. The child's clothing, towels, bedding, hairbrushes, combs, barrettes, curlers, and head gear should be boiled. If an item cannot be boiled, it should be washed in the hottest water possible and then ironed. Dry-cleaning is also effective.

Limping

If limited movement of the hip, knee, or ankle persists for more than a couple of days and cannot be easily connected to an obvious injury, the child should be evaluated by a physician. The limping may reflect a problem in the joint being favored, but in some cases it may be caused by a tumor or injury of the bone shaft or muscle or by an orthopedic problem that requires treatment. Any child who is limping and has a fever should be seen by a physician immediately.

M

Masturbation

Self-exploration is part of children's normal curiosity about their own bodies. Once they find that handling their genitals is pleasurable, they then masturbate because it feels good. This self-manipulation of their genitals for sexual excitation or gratification is normal; it may even enhance their sex lives once they become adults.

Parents should not express concern, nor should they try to shame children or frighten them by telling myths about a part falling off, or hair growing on one's hands, or other falsehoods that were often related in more repressive eras. Properly approached, masturbation becomes just a small part of a child's overall experience and no difficulties arise from it.

However, compulsive masturbation is often a means of releasing tensions accumulating because of an emotional problem, marital tension in the child's family, undue sibling rivalry, or a feeling of rejection by peers or family members. In children who are affected, masturbation may occur with extreme frequency, conspicuously, and at inappropriate times and places. If the parents become upset and punitive, the situation seems to worsen. Hence, evaluation by a professional is advised.

Menstrual Difficulties

Disorders of menstruation, such as delayed onset, abnormal bleeding, and excessive pain, are not uncommon in adolescent girls. Extremely complex hormonal and anatomical processes are involved, and it normally takes some time for these systems to function smoothly and regularly.

Parents should be sure that their daughters know about menstruation before it occurs. A good time may be when the girl first starts to show physical signs of sexual development (breast buds), although younger children may express interest in the subject. Several pamphlets and books are available that explain the process in understandable language. But nothing is quite so comforting as a personal talk in which the normality of menstrual bleeding is stressed and girls are encouraged to regard this as a sign of growing maturity rather than a nuisance. Most frequently, girls prefer to talk with their mothers or other female caretakers, since they are often embarrassed about sex and may feel more comfortable talking with a woman.

Cramping, abdominal discomfort, backache, and leg aches are common complaints. Tension aggravates these symptoms, and severe anxiety about menstruation may result in vomiting, paleness, and occasional fainting. If school attendance or other activities are interrupted, medications are available, but it is advisable that the girl consult with her doctor so that the situation can be evaluated and an appropriate prescription obtained.

Parents should be reassured that it may take several months for a regular menstrual pattern to become established. Bleeding may be spotty one time and normal the next. Sometimes as long as six months may elapse between periods. Excessive or prolonged flow (lasting more than a week) should be reported to the girl's doctor or health-care professional.

Most girls in the United States start their periods at around 12 years of age. Only if the delay goes beyond 16 need a doctor be consulted, unless other symptoms are present.

Far more often than not, teenagers' menstrual difficulties clear up of their own accord. However, if discomfort remains severe, irregularity continues, bleeding is heavy and prolonged, or there is an excessive delay in menarche (onset of menstruation), the young girl should definitely see her doctor or health-care professional. Possible causes of abnormal menstrual difficulties include conditions that affect the hypothalamus or the thyroid gland, nutritional deficits, emotional stress, chromosomal and endocrine disorders, as well as the use of certain drugs that may have been prescribed for other conditions.

Mental Retardation

Causes of mental retardation — delayed development in language, social, and adaptive skills so that the child fails to reach the level of functioning appropriate for his or her age — are varied, and include:

- Genetic factors, usually with a family history of prior mental retardation
- Chromosomal and metabolic abnormalities
- Prenatal or at-birth infections
- Maternal drug abuse
- Injuries

However, medical experts estimate that in approximately 80 percent of cases, the cause cannot be determined.

Parents of a mentally retarded child should know their child's category of retardation so they can have some input into determining the most appropriate learning environment and how best to structure the home environment if the child is to continue living with the family.

Psychological evaluation is essential. According to the child's age, the most popular tests, listed below in ascending order of age use (from under 2 to 15 years and 11 months), are the Bayley Scale of Infant Development, the Stanford-Binet, the Wechsler Preschool and Primary Scale of Intelligence, and the Wechsler Intelligence Scale for Children. For children up to 5 years, the Denver Developmental Screening Test provides some approximation of intelligence level. The categories of retardation are:

- *Borderline children* (*IQ 84 to 71*). These children have trouble learning in a regular school. But once out of school, they tend to blend into the general population. They can support themselves at jobs that are not too demanding. Approximately 14 percent of all children tested in schools are in this group.
- *Mildly retarded children* (*IQ 70 to 50*). Such children are termed "educable." Some of them can be taught to read up to a fourth- to sixth-grade level, so many of them can be expected to be self-supporting in menial jobs.
- *Moderately retarded children* (*IQ 49 to 35*). Such children are termed "trainable." That is, they can generally be expected to take care of their personal needs of dressing, washing, eating, and the like, and they may gather some minimal social skills. But they generally always require a structured, supportive environment. Partly because of obvious language and motor impairments, and partly because their thinking is so concrete and childlike, they are apt to experience considerable trouble dealing with the outside world.

- *Severely retarded children (IQ 34 to 20)*. These children are somewhat trainable, but to a far lesser degree than the moderately retarded. Therefore, they require a highly supervised, structured environment.
- *Profoundly retarded children (IQ 19 and below)*. These children usually cannot even learn to walk, let alone talk. Vocalizations are usually confined to unintelligible grunts, and it is totally unreasonable to expect such a child to attain any degree of self-sufficiency.

Parents should also be aware of the fact that, just as with children who have normal intelligence or higher, mental illness can occur in the mentally retarded. It may be harder to diagnose and treat because of the child's limited verbal skills; however, it may manifest itself in many ways, including destructive behavior disorders.

Once the degree of retardation is established, the child's parents, and any siblings, should consult with appropriate specialists who can assist them in making decisions about the child's home setting, educational programs, and the setting of realistic goals for everyone involved. Genetic counseling may also be useful if the mental retardation is thought or known to be hereditary.

For more information, call the toll-free number of the American Association of Mentally Retarded, 800-424-3688.

Migraine

See HEADACHE

Moodiness

Depending on various factors behind this behavior, in which children or adolescents generally become quiet and avoid interacting with people around them, the withdrawal may last only a day or two, with an abrupt return to normal. At times mood swings, from very sad to very joyful, may be quite wide and quite prolonged.

Adolescents are especially given to wide mood swings. From an adult's viewpoint, these periods of moodiness may seem inappropriate in the context of what is really happening. A 16-year-old may be bouncy and cheerful as he leaves for school, even though rain is pouring down, his best friend just moved away, and he failed an important examination. The next day may be bright and sunny, his best friend calls to invite him for a long weekend, and he gets an A in an even more important exam, but this same teenager snaps at every-one all during dinner and then retires to his room to listen to the stereo and stare off into space.

It is not as important to understand such behavior as it is to *accept* it as normal.

Preadolescents generally tend to be much less moody. If moodiness does occur, it is most likely a reaction to stress at school, with peers, or other family members, and it does not last long.

Of course, if the child or adolescent seems to have unusually long or severe bouts of moodiness, or when symptoms of DEPRESSION seem to be present and parents cannot discover a source or a solution in a supportive, nonconfrontational discussion, it may be wise to seek professional help.

Muscle Weakness

Some families have a rare genetic disorder in which periodic episodes of muscle weakness occur. This disorder, called *familial periodic paralysis*, was formerly considered essentially untreatable, aside from resting after an attack. Currently, doctors prescribe oral potassium chloride and acetazolamide for control of symptoms.

MUSCULAR DYSTROPHY is a disease in which muscle weakness is the predominant feature. An untreated THYROID DISORDER, either hyper- or hypothyroidism, can also cause muscle weakness.

Because muscle weakness, sometimes accompanied by muscle pain, may indicate a serious disorder, parents are advised to arrange for a medical evaluation whenever a child shows any signs of weakness, such as difficulty climbing stairs, getting up from a sitting position, or an unusual manner of walking.

N

Nail Biting

Biting is considered by most mental-health authorities to be a sign of aggression. Often very young children bite their nails in an effort to control acts of aggression they may not want to direct outward. Nail biting may also offer a child something to do when the environment is not very stimulating or when he or she would rather be screaming but subconsciously senses that chewing is the wiser choice. Whatever the origin, nail biting eventually becomes a habit.

Parents should not scold or punish the child. Many children outgrow the habit when they learn to care about their own appearance. Also, if it is done in private and is not so extensive as to resemble anything more than a very close clipping, it may be best to ignore the situation. However, if the nail biting is severe enough to prohibit normal nail growth, causes small skin breaks that can become infected, or the child bites the nails compulsively, then some steps should be taken.

On occasion, the unraveling of some stressful problem enables the child to stop nail biting. More often than not, a direct behavioral therapy approach works best. Try establishing a schedule in which the child may chew all the nails *except* the pinkies for a period of two weeks, at which time some definite, preset reward will be given. Next, the child may bite all the nails except the pinkies and the ring fingers, again with a reward in mind. Repeat this until all the fingers have been eliminated as chewable. During all this time, a substitute chewable such as sugarless gum or mints might be offered.

Parents should be patient. The biting became a habit slowly, and so will the nonbiting. Only if severe nail biting is accompanied by other signs of undue stress, such as EMOTIONAL WITHDRAWAL or very easily aroused anger, need professional advice be sought.

Nails, Problems with

For the first several months of life, babies' nails are soft and pliable, often splitting before attaining much length. If cutting is needed, parents should be careful not to cut too close to the fingertips. Rounding with a soft emery board is even better, since clipping could accidentally break the skin and provide an easy route for infection. Toenails should be cut straight across and with enough length left so that nail margins extend slightly beyond the soft tissues of the toe. This method avoids ingrown toenails, especially as the child begins to walk and wear shoes.

Some teenage girls complain of fingernail splitting, which is caused by brittleness. Although there may be some underlying abnormality of nail structure, the problem is aggravated by filing, by using nail-polish removers, and by too frequent contact with soap and water. Treatment includes applying hand creams around the nail bed, gentle manicuring, and, if the girl chooses, several layers of polish to discourage splitting.

Paronychia (infections around the nail bed) may occur and must be treated by a physician. Antibiotics are prescribed, and if soaking according to the doctor's suggestion does not allow for proper draining, surgical drainage may have to be done.

Injury to nails may cause a whitish discoloration or a collection of blood beneath the affected nail. The pain may be extremely intense, even though the injury cannot be classified as dangerous. Again, medical help should be sought; the doctor may shave the nail or release the pressure by applying heated metal.

When an injury causes loss of a nail, parents and the child need to be patient. It takes a fingernail some three to six months and a toenail some six to eight months to grow back.

Nails also serve as a clue to general health. Bluish nails may signal some heart or blood-vascular disorder. Pale nails may be present in ANEMIA. Nutritional deficits may also be signaled by discoloration of the nails, and certain deformities, such as ridges or pitting, may indicate other generalized disease, sometimes of a congenital (present-at-birth) nature. If parents note any of these abnormalities, they should speak with a doctor or other health-care professional and arrange a medical examination for the child.

Nervousness

This is a general term for an uneasy and/or agitated emotional state that can be behaviorally indicated by fidgeting, physiologically expressed by signs such as a fast pulse rate, and caused by factors ranging from a THYROID DISORDER such as an overactive thyroid gland to the presence of an ATTENTION-DEFICIT DISORDER.

However, more often than not, nervousness is simply a transient sense of uneasiness such as adults feel from time to time. Only when the frequency and degree seem grossly out of proportion to what is occurring around the child should parents be concerned. If supportive and reassuring discussion fails to reveal a cause and suggest a solution, it may be best to consult with a mental-health professional once the child's doctor or health-care professional rules out any physical cause.

Nightmares and Night Terrors

Sleep allows children to experience their own unconscious minds in a direct and uncensored way. Day-to-day happenings may be lived out in ways that cannot be perceived consciously or intellectually, and this relates very much to the child's level of cognitive and social development.

Children may not be able to even recognize, let alone discuss, fearful stresses such as new situations, school changes, dimly perceived family problems (for example, financial strain), or difficulties with friends.

Occasional nightmares and night terrors are rather common in children between the ages of four and eight, probably for the reasons mentioned above. An episode of nightmare is rather fleeting, and sometimes children can tell their parents about the dream. In the case of night terror, children may not quite awaken completely for a period of time, yet they cry out, look quite terrified, and may thrash about. They remain in what psychiatrists term a "twilight state," showing the appearance of experiencing great terror, still "seeing" frightening things, and not responding to the parents. Once awake, they may not remember at all what they were thinking while asleep.

Holding and reassuring the child usually provide sufficient comfort. If the child seems fearful of the dark, keeping a night-light on may offer further solace. Children should remain in their own beds; they should *not* be allowed to sleep with their parents, which would reinforce the notion that something is unsafe and would also contribute to an unfortunate behavior pattern that may become difficult to change. Parents should *never* chase imaginary bears out of a closet or close shutters so ghosts cannot come in the window. This only confuses children further, increasing the difficulty in differentiating reality from fantasy and making them wonder if, indeed, terrifying night creatures actually do exist.

Other children, particularly adolescents, can be expected to have nightmares that exaggerate their daytime worries of losing the next football game, missing a prom, failing an examination, or losing the affection of a sibling or parent. Because of their greater cognitive and social development, adolescents usually have little trouble recognizing nightmares for what they are: nightmares. They may even take some emotional comfort and some intellectual stimulation in discussing these dreams and analyzing what they represent.

Of course, if family tensions are the root of the night terrors, counseling may be a way of working out the problems and ending the nighttime activities.

O

Obesity

See WEIGHT GAIN

P

Palpitation

The sensation of a throbbing, fluttering, or pulsating heart is often associated with an unusually rapid heart rate. It generally lasts only a short time (usually a few seconds) and is ordinarily no cause for alarm. Sometimes palpitations can be a side effect of either a prescription or nonprescription drug.

If the condition persists, happens quite frequently, or worries the child, parents should arrange for a medical examination. In almost all cases palpitations will be tagged "functional," that is, having no organic or disease-related basis.

Penis Swelling

Swelling may result from a bruise or bump against a hard object, such as might occur in a bicycle accident. Younger boys sometimes sustain a so-called ammonia burn from wet diapers or underclothing that may cause swelling. Healing and the prevention of further episodes are achieved by applying a protective cream or ointment as recommended by the local pharmacist or the family doctor or health-care professional.

Severe swelling of the penis, as well as a number of other abnormalities, such as *phimosis* (an inflammatory constriction of the foreskin) or defects in the urinary opening, demand prompt medical evaluation and treatment.

If the foreskin is tight and retracted back over the head of the penis, a compression may occur that causes considerable swelling and pain. Soaking the penis in warm saltwater may help reduce the swelling so that the foreskin can be gradually drawn forward.

Physical Disability

Children handle their physical disabilities precisely the way their parents handle them. If children are considered handicapped, they

255

will consider themselves handicapped and increasingly refuse to try to do things that, with a little patience, they can learn to do.

If physically disabled children are reassured of their worth and receive consistently loving encouragement, they may find new ways to work around their limitations. Emotional support is also valuable in compensating for teasing by other children; it may even stop or prevent such teasing if the disabled child's conduct is self-assured.

Poisoning

Youngsters who have accidentally poisoned themselves can often be saved by prompt first aid. Adolescents who have taken poison in a suicide gesture or attempt, or who have overdosed on illicit or even legal drugs, may be expected to be uncooperative. Parents should not hesitate to call the police for help, in addition to contacting an emergency treatment facility.

Parents should always have a bottle of syrup of ipecac (available at the local pharmacy) on hand. Activated charcoal liquid is also a useful antidote to many poisons. Some manufacturers have devised antipoison kits that contain measured doses of antidotes, along with specific instructions. Consider purchasing these kits, and keep this material readily available.

Also, fill in the important phone numbers on the lines provided in the front of this book, and keep a second list by the phone.

In most instances of childhood poisoning, *prevention* is the key. Parents should take care to childproof their home by keeping dangerous cleaning fluids or powders, plumbing solutions, and other such materials in safe places where curious youngsters cannot find them. Parents should also remember that many substances not generally thought of as being poisonous can readily poison a youngster who consumes too much. These substances include ordinary aspirin and other nonprescription painkillers.

In the unfortunate instance that all childproofing precautions are to no avail and an accidental poisoning occurs, *call the poison-control center or the child's doctor for advice about what first-aid measures can be undertaken safely. Then immediately call for emergency medical assistance.* When there is another adult or a responsible older child at home at the time, this person should do the calling while the other performs first-aid measures.

If the child or adolescent is unconscious, there is nothing to do — that is, nothing you *should* do — until trained personnel arrive. On the other hand, if the child is conscious and vomiting must be induced or choking suppressed, here are some directions. If the child is not breathing but there is a pulse, perform some type of artificial respiration.

The following instructions are meant only as a brief guide to first aid. *REMEMBER:* Time is important! Getting professional help is important!

- *Vomiting.* If the child has taken lye or some other strong alkali, strong acids, cleaning fluid, or petroleum distillates such as kerosene, gasoline, coal oil, fuel oil, or paint thinner, do *not* attempt to induce vomiting unless the poison-control center, doctor, or other authority advises it.

  If vomiting is indicated, follow these instructions: Mix one tablepoon (½ ounce) syrup of ipecac with one cup water. (Do not use a salt-and-water solution.) Have the child drink this as quickly as possible, until vomiting occurs. Keep the child facedown with the head lower than the hips to prevent choking while vomiting. If no vomiting occurs within 20 minutes after the syrup of ipecac is given, repeat the same dose — but only once. See that a sample of the vomitus is kept for examination. When the child is transported to a medical facility, take along the poison container, with its label intact.
- *Choking. See* CHOKING
- *Artificial respiration.* For the mouth-to-mouth or mouth-to-nose technique, clear the child's mouth with your fingers only if necessary. With the child lying down on his or her back, tilt the head back and breathe directly into the mouth or nose until you see the chest rise. Then remove your mouth from the child's, allowing the lungs to empty. Keep repeating this at the rate of about 20 times each minute. If the victim is an infant, breathe shallow little puffs of air. Cardiopulmonary resuscitation (CPR) or external cardiac compression should be carried out simultaneously by another adult or older child who has been trained in the technique. The American Red Cross and other organizations frequently give training sessions for the general public, and both parents should know how to perform this lifesaving procedure.

Prematurity

An infant born before full development within the uterus — which usually takes 40 weeks or 9 lunar months — is said to be premature.

Before birth, special medical techniques such as ultrasound (a special kind of x-ray-type examination that measures sound waves) and amniocentesis (withdrawing and analyzing some amniotic fluid) may help to determine the infant's level of maturity. A fluid specimen withdrawn from the uterus may, for example, be tested to see if the baby's lungs are developed enough to allow survival without special respiratory-therapy measures. Generally speaking, however, examination after birth is the best guide to assessing the premature infant's level of development.

All the important organs are basically formed by the sixth month of pregnancy, but they need more time to complete development. Premature babies have small stomachs, and they suck and swallow poorly. Their lungs need to be stronger, and they are especially prone to infections because their antibodies are not ready to defend them. The first 24 to 48 hours are the most crucial. The longer the pregnancy, the better the baby's chances for survival.

If the baby is more than five pounds, he or she may not need to be placed in an incubator. Smaller infants, however, usually are. In the incubator, the baby's surroundings can be maintained much as they were in the mother's uterus, and because of the glass and plastic sides, doctors and nurses can keep a close watch. Premature infants may be given oxygen and fed by tube. In this special setting, they can be weighed (a good key to whether the child is thriving), bathed, diapered, and otherwise taken care of.

As a rule of thumb, if a premature infant is born at 2 pounds, he or she is kept in the hospital for two months. Babies are generally discharged when they weigh about 5½ pounds.

Once home, a premature baby needs to be fed more often than a full-term baby, and the doctor may suggest vitamins and an iron formula. The nursery should be kept warmer than usual. Visits to the doctor may also be made more frequently than usual, possibly as often as every ten days for whatever period of time the doctor advises.

Parents of premature infants should not consider these children particularly fragile or in any way hampered. As the baby grows, he or she will catch up in terms of both size and general development. In the last 25 years, great strides have been made in the care of premature infants. An entire specialty — neonatology — has introduced highly specialized techniques and very sophisticated equipment into the prebirth, newborn, and early-infancy care of premature babies.

R

Regressive Behavior

This is behavior in which a child goes back (to activities characteristic of a younger age, for example, a five-year-old starting to suck his thumb or wet his pants, or a four-year-old reverting to the baby talk she outgrew two years earlier.

Usually such behavior is a coping mechanism, a means of dealing with stress experienced at the arrival of a new baby, the family's move to a new location, or some other factor that observant parents can usually deduce. Generally speaking, parents are better off ignoring this temporary change in behavior. Scolding or mocking the child — for example, by making remarks such as, "My, I thought you were 4½, not a baby" — may act to reinforce the behavior as an attention-getting device.

If, however, the source of the child's stress cannot be determined and the regressive behavior continues longer than a week or two, parents may wish to seek professional advice, especially if the child also shows signs of EMOTIONAL WITHDRAWAL or DEPRESSION.

Restless Behavior

This involves constant moving around or fidgeting, or a sleep disturbance usually induced by overexcitement or the experience of stress.

Boredom or the desire to be doing something else makes even the healthiest child restless, a phenomenon especially noticeable on rainy days or when children are almost but not quite recovered from an illness.

Only when restless behavior is associated with impulsivity, a short ATTENTION SPAN, and extreme hyperactivity need parents suspect a possible ATTENTION-DEFICIT DISORDER that demands professional assessment.

Rocking

This rhythmic movement in which an infant or young child rocks to and fro, especially before going to sleep, seems to induce relaxation, although at times it may become quite forceful and include HEAD BANGING.

Many children who rock excessively seem to be more easily agitated by noise and movement around them than other children are. Cutting down on these stimuli may decrease the rocking. Older children engage in this behavior less often if they are allowed to do it by more socially appropriate means, as in a small rocking chair.

S

Scars

Scars appear anywhere on or in the body, but the tendency is to think in terms of skin wounds.

Depending on the extent of the injury, scar formation may take many months, and the tissue changes appearance several times. At first the injured area appears reddened and the scar line seems relatively wide. Gradually the area whitens as the tissue under the injury builds strength. Eventually the rough and uneven surface draws back, and the scar assumes its true size and color.

Children are especially prone to many accidents that leave scars, especially around the knees, legs, and, to a somewhat lesser extent, arms. Faces, heads, and lips are not immune, although modern techniques of clamping or suturing may make such scars almost invisible.

Unless scars are genuinely disfiguring, they should probably be ignored.

Sexual Abuse, Molestation

The child who has been sexually abused undergoes special trauma because sexuality is undefined, poorly understood, confusing, and often scary.

Parents may compound this problem and unwittingly contribute to the potential for hampered sexual maturing by too loudly expressing their anger, fear, distaste, and vindictiveness toward the guilty party. An air of calm and support should prevail, especially when reporting the crime and during the offender's prosecution. The parents and child may find themselves walking an emotional tightrope after the attack. To help the child avoid dwelling on the event, parents and others should not dwell upon it, especially in the child's presence. However, the event should not be ignored. Allow the child to talk about the incident when he or she wishes. To avoid emotional difficulties, the child needs supportive counseling by professionals who specialize in working with victims of sexual abuse.

Sexual Development, Premature

Hormonal changes at puberty cause the development of what are termed secondary sexual characteristics: male or female distribution of body hair; breast enlargement in the female; enlargement of the testicles and penis as well as voice changes in the male.

On occasion, signs of secondary development may be noticed in very young children. A two- or three-year-old girl may show breast enlargement. A little boy may develop pubic and armpit hair without showing any growth in the size of testicles. Secondary sexual characteristics can be considered premature if they occur in a girl younger than 8½ or a boy younger than 10 — approximately three years earlier than the average ages at which such changes occur.

The situation arises because of premature production of hormones in the brain, the ovaries or testes, adrenal glands, and, in a few cases, the liver. The changes are essentially harmless, but the child certainly should be evaluated by a physician to make sure there is no underlying disease contributing to the early development.

Parents should remember that from the age of 8 or 10 well into adolescence, children want very much to be like their peers. Thus a boy in intermediate school may be more embarrassed by than proud of his bass voice. At times, professional counseling may be needed if the child becomes unduly disturbed by these bodily changes.

Sexual Preoccupation

Inordinate attention to sexual matters usually stems from anxiety about sex. It may stem from entirely different matters, but most authorities believe it is stimulated by viewing explicit sexual material, observing parents or other adults during intercourse, or witnessing nudity in the household.

Children are quite normally curious about sex and their own sexual feelings, but facing these issues before they are sufficiently mature may cause considerable confusion and emotional discomfort. Instead of running from the subject, some children become fascinated, further stimulated, and then quite preoccupied. They should not be teased or punished, but they should be encouraged to discuss their feelings and their fears on whatever level the *child* indicates is comfortable. If the problem cannot be solved at home, the parents and the child may benefit from some professional counseling.

Sibling Rivalry

There is nothing unusual or potentially disastrous about the struggle that may go on among brothers and sisters jockeying to be the sole recipient of the love, attention, and approval of one or both parents, which has come to be known as sibling rivalry. But this normal developmental stage is, nonetheless, disturbing to many parents, who think that something must be wrong with their children or that they are parenting incorrectly.

Part of the problem is that most parents can't observe how other families' children behave in similar situations. Parents, who see only their own children behind closed doors, tend to think their kids fight more than other children, who always seem so well behaved. But what is happening in the privacy of your home is probably happening in the privacy of others, and other parents probably are wishing their children behaved as well as yours do.

It's only natural that children who spend so much time together will find ways to get on each other's nerves. Many psychologists believe that the rivalry is a good thing (though not to be encouraged or promoted), and that the competitiveness can transform into ways of coping better with the world — and the other sibling — as a grownup. But for that to happen, the parent has to be able to help the children channel that rivalry into productive areas.

One thing to do when things get out of hand is to step in and stop the fighting, but try not to play favorites (and, especially, gender favorites), or constantly compare one child's behavior favorably to another's failings. Do what has to be done to maintain order and house rules and use the opportunity to teach important social lessons. The loud spats of sibling rivalry don't have to be destructive — they can be very constructive.

Some psychologists feel that the age difference between the two children may be a factor in the existence or intensity of the rivalry. The toddler feels jealous of a new intruder taking the mother's attention away — attention he or she "deserves." Many experts feel that if you are planning a family, a gap of about three years between children may minimize later sibling rivalry.

But it may be that nothing you do can stop the fighting, or that you feel inadequate to cope with the problem. You might find some ideas and tactics in books about sibling rivalry. Then again, you may need to consider bringing in professional help, such as a specialist in child psychology. You may also have to face up to the fact that, even though you have done nothing wrong, your children may have rivalries that last their entire lifetimes. But most siblings do outgrow the rivalry.

Sleep Problems

Falling under the umbrella term *insomnia*, disturbances of the normal sleep process involve the inability to get to sleep, constant awakening, getting out of bed and wandering about, and difficulty falling back to sleep.

Most sleep problems in children can be prevented by consistent behavior on the part of the parents. Bedtimes should be established and followed. Certain bedtime rituals may help: tucking in, bedtime stories, a brief conversation about the day's events, or, for babies, some gentle patting.

Sleepwalking

This is a sleep disturbance in which the child walks around even though he or she is not alert or fully awake, and it is somewhat more common in boys than in girls. The fact that it is frequently outgrown suggests more of a maturational than an emotional basis.

Parents may wish to take precautions around the house such as installing a gate at the tops of stairways in multilevel homes and being sure that windows and exterior doors are locked. The child's bedroom door should *never* be locked from the outside in case of fire or some other emergency. A screen door may be trimmed to fit the child's bedroom door, which will allow parents to look in and the child to look out or call out and be heard if need be while acting as a barrier.

Although sleepwalking is usually harmless and, incredibly, most children do not hurt themselves while in this state, the phenomenon can on occasion signal some psychiatric or medical difficulty. So if the problem persists over a long period of time or the child shows evidence of other problems, he or she should be checked by a qualified professional.

See also NIGHTMARES AND NIGHT TERROR

Smoking

Even though cigarette smoking is a habit on the decline in the United States, teenagers and preteens can still be expected to try it, especially if they are told not to or that it is not good for them — rebellion and the need to feel independent are natural young-adult urges. It is especially difficult to keep them from smoking when they see their favorite movie stars lighting up in films, or when they note that glamorous sporting events or their favorite musical performers' national tours are sponsored by cigarette companies. A cigarette can seem like a very "cool" prop.

The long-term health threats of smoking — lung cancer and emphysema, among others — mean little to youngsters, who think they are immortal and indestructible. A better approach might be to emphasize self-image: Remind the teen or preteen that smoking makes their clothes and breath smell bad and their teeth yellow, and makes them cough unpleasantly too much of the time — very "uncool" to people they want to impress, such as certain members of the opposite sex.

There is another smoking problem. Recent studies show that "passive smoking" — simply breathing the tobacco smoke that is in the air in a room — is a significant health hazard responsible for thousands of deaths a year. And it is especially dangerous for children, possibly leading to the development of heart disease and to almost 20 percent of all lung cancer cases among nonsmokers. Young people, as much as possible, should be in smoke-free environments. Parents and other adult role models should avoid smoking, and certainly should not smoke in the presence of children.

Snoring

Snoring is caused by the soft palate (spongy tissue toward the back of the roof of the mouth) vibrating during sleep with the mouth open. Snoring is usually not of any great medical importance. It may result simply from the nasal congestion that usually accompanies a cold. However, children who habitually breathe through the mouth should be checked by their doctor or health-care professional to see whether they are suffering from enlarged adenoids.

See TONSILLITIS

Sore Throat

Inflammation of the throat, medically known as pharyngitis, is extremely common throughout the childhood years.

Most sore throats occur because of minor viral infections such as the common cold with nasal congestion, and they usually clear up in a day or two if the child is given plenty of fluids. Allowing a child to use a straw may encourage frequent drinking. A child who can gargle can do so as often as it seems necessary to relieve the pain: saltwater solutions (½ teaspoon salt in 8 ounces of water) or strong tea (either hot or cold) may be used.

However, parents should be alert to the possibility of a streptococcus, or "strep," infection. The only way to make sure a strep infection exists is for the doctor to swab the back of the throat and then culture the specimen to see if it contains strep germs. If it does, then the child is given antibiotics, largely in an effort to prevent RHEUMATIC FEVER. Even if the child feels better and the sore throat goes away, antibiotic therapy should be continued for whatever period the doctor prescribes. Some physicians will, once the therapy is stopped, take another throat culture to make certain the streptococci germs are gone.

Sometimes a child with an inflammation of the thyroid gland may complain of a burning in the neck and throat, but on medical examination the throat appears normal.

When parents are in doubt, or the child seems to have sore throats more often than most children — especially when FEVER is present — the safest choice is to have the child examined by his or her doctor, for sore throat can be a symptom of many disorders.

See also ALLERGIES, BACTERIAL INFECTIONS, CHICKENPOX, CROUP, HERPANGINA, HERPETIC STOMATITIS, INFECTIOUS MONONUCLEOSIS, MEASLES, RUBELLA, SCARLET FEVER, TONSILLITIS

Speech, Delayed

Although there are no hard-and-fast rules about when intelligible speech should be expected, most children are able to speak a few words by the time they are two years old and a complete sentence or two by the time they reach age three.

Results of many studies show that when parents consistently talk to their infants using real words and complete sentences rather than baby talk, read to them, and conduct normal conversations in their presence, babies learn to speak at an earlier age. On the other hand, some perfectly normal and even exceptionally bright children seem to prefer not to talk when they are supposed to; frequently, these same children begin to speak in complete, well-structured, and cogent sentences when they are three or four years old.

The great leap in language development occurs from the ages of two to five, with general fluency being achieved by the time the child is six.

Again, parents desperate to hear their first "mama" and "dada" should be reassured that speech patterns are highly individual; if their child seems slow, they should not worry unduly. Of course, if a two-year-old child cannot communicate even the simplest words, a medical evaluation is in order to make sure the toddler is not suffering from a HEARING LOSS or congenital (present-at-birth) DEAFNESS. Some children may have the ability to hear everything said to them (receptive language), but an inability to state their responses or anything else (expressive language). Speech therapy might help the child break the ice and make some speech strides. Check first with the local school system to see if testing is done and special preschool classes are offered.

See also STUTTERING; SPEECH in Appendix I: Norms and Values

Spitting Up

This regurgitation of milk drunk by infants differs from vomiting in that it is not forceful — fluids tend simply to dribble out of the mouth and onto the chin. It may occur just after a feeding or as long as two hours later, in which case the fluid may be sour, because of the actions of digestive acids on the milk.

As long as the infant is thriving and there is no true vomiting, spitting up is more of a nuisance than a serious problem. Keeping the baby somewhat upright for 20 minutes after each feeding may lessen spitting up. Careful attention should also be paid to the amount of milk given, since overfeeding increases the problem. Parents should also avoid vigorous handling or play right after the baby is fed.

If the spitting up continues to present a problem, the child's doctor or health-care professional may recommend a cereal-thickened formula.

Compare PYLORIC STENOSIS

Staggering

See FALLING, MUSCLE WEAKNESS

Stammering

See STUTTERING

Staring Spells

Daydreaming or boredom can account for these brief episodes in which a child seems to lose contact with his or her surroundings. Staring spells are most common in four- to eight-year-old children with active imaginations. Recurrent and/or very frequent staring spells may, however, be part of a SEIZURE DISORDER called *petit mal syndrome.* Therefore, parents should be alert to a possible need for medical evaluation so that any underlying disorder can be treated.

Stomachache

See ABDOMINAL PAIN

Strangers, Fear of

This phenomenon — characterized by normal infants' screaming and strong attempts to avoid contact with anyone except parents or daily caretakers — is caused by the emergence of what psychologists and other professionals call "object identity." By the age of two or three months, most infants have a sense of object permanence, the concept that people and other objects continue to exist even when, for the moment, they cannot be seen, touched, or heard. At about six months babies begin to develop the sense of object identity, by which they are able to sense the unique qualities of themselves and others around them. However, they still feel a strong attachment to their mothers, since, at an earlier stage, they could not really differentiate themselves and their mothers as being separate. This growing individualization, combined with a strong tie to their mothers, sometimes causes a discomforting anxiety.

It is at this time that babies who at one point could be left with just about anybody start to protest loudly when left alone with strangers, even grandparents or other relatives and friends they have seen before. By the time the child is about one year old, he or she has learned to discriminate more finely between one person and the next, is more certain that the disappeared mother or other caretaker will return, and is comfortable with an increasing number of different people after a brief period of getting acquainted. Between the ages of one and two, as children acquire more and more autonomy, they are able to tolerate increasingly longer separations from their mothers in the company of others. Some children may at that time become a little shy when confronted by people entirely new to them, but this differs from stranger fear and it, too, is a stage that is normally outgrown within a few months.

Stuttering

During the usual period of rapid language development, between the ages of two and five, nearly all children pause, block, and repeat sounds. No one knows exactly why this is so, but an interesting theory has been advanced. It is thought that although young children understand language and may understand rudimentary rules for sentence structure, sometimes of their own making, they simply lack practice in fluent speech. Therefore the natural flow of sentences gets blocked and, in their effort to overcome any lack of clarity, children's speech may become even less fluent.

If parents or older siblings avoid eye contact or overreact by telling the child to think first, speak more slowly, start all over again, and so on, the child may turn this negative reaction inward, heightening self-consciousness about speaking.

Thus, family interaction may be a key factor that leads to psychological difficulties that reinforce the problem. In only the rarest of instances is there any neurological component, and there is no evidence that stuttering is hereditary or even that children learn to stutter by imitating poor speech patterns.

If noninterference remains standard — for example, not interrupting or making demands — and if all the family carefully avoids teasing, then the child who stutters for more than a few months during this language-development phase should be taken for experienced professional evaluation. After ruling out HEARING LOSS or DEAFNESS, the doctor may recommend the services of a qualified speech therapist.

Even highly verbal, extremely fluent speakers sometimes stutter if they are overly excited or embarrassed. Therefore, temporary spells of such stammering by children should be overlooked.

For more information, call the Stuttering Hot Line of the National Center for Stuttering, 800-221-2483 (212-532-1460 in New York City).

Suicide

The subject of suicide makes many people extremely uncomfortable, especially when parents must confront the cold fact that suicide is now a leading cause of death in teenagers, rated second or third in some studies. Between 1950 and 1975, the incidence of adolescent suicide tripled, and the rate continues to rise. This is especially significant because a death is generally not listed as suicide unless there is proof of intention to commit suicide, such as prior threats, suicidal gestures such as unsuccessful previous attempts, or a note or statement. Other suicide statistics:

- Suicides have tripled among 10- to 14-year-olds over the last two decades; among 15- to 19-year-olds, the incidence has doubled.
- Whites are three times as likely to kill themselves as are blacks.
- Adolescent girls try to kill themselves four to five times more often than boys, but the boys are more likely to succeed (probably because they select more thorough, lethal methods — boys choose guns or hanging, while girls opt for pills).

Many parents wrongfully assume that their own adolescent problems can be equated with those teenagers face today. With continuing threats of nuclear holocaust, increasing high technology that imposes ever-mounting demands on youngsters trying to make up their minds about what to do with their lives, and widespread turbulence in people's convictions about many traditional values, each new generation faces more complex problems. When this unrest is coupled with the physical and emotional development adolescents face, some of them decide they can no longer cope with life and the only way out is death.

If parents are able to recognize the seriousness of their child's plight and sincerely show loving concern, the adolescent may reach a new level of maturity in which other alternatives become more attractive. This is especially true when, after a suicidal gesture, the teenager realizes that he or she need not go to such extremes to get attention and respect. At the same time, parents must know that attention, respect, love, and concern *in advance* do not, unfortunately, always ensure against teenagers attempting suicide.

The old advice about ignoring suicide threats and the old saying that people who talk about committing suicide do not do it are totally wrong. Suicidal talk and suicidal gestures are serious cries for help. Such youngsters need counseling with a professional who is experienced with such cases and with whom the teenager can develop a viable and trusting relationship. Concurrent family therapy may be advisable, not only as an acknowledgment of the whole family's interest and support and as a means by which the teenager can express his or her feelings in neutral surroundings, but also so that the rest of the family can learn how their own conflicts may be contributing to the child's dilemma. Some restructuring of the home environment may be in order.

School truancy, SLEEP PROBLEMS, preoccupation with bodily health, vague physical symptoms (particularly unexplained HEADACHE or AB-DOMINAL PAIN), DEPRESSION, EMOTIONAL WITHDRAWAL, weight loss, irritability, ADDICTION to alcohol or drugs, and running away from home are all signs that studies have shown may indicate escape behavior that may lead to suicide.

Parents should heed these kinds of warnings and ask for professional help. Denying the problem will not make it go away, and long-term follow-ups of would-be adolescent suicides show that most become healthy and productive adults.

Unfortunately, there are times that even the strongest efforts fail and determined children succeed in killing themselves. Trying to relive the past and the whole sequence of events is an unavoidable parental reaction. Parents going through this extremely painful period of bereavement should seek professional help and continue with counseling until they have come to terms with the loss and their own guilt feelings.

T

Teeth, Order of Appearance

Some parents believe that a child's first teeth need to appear in a certain order — usually bottom front two, top front two, and then the two on either side of those — and that any other order of appearance of the teeth is abnormal and something to be concerned about. Nothing could be farther from the truth. Though many children may manifest their first teeth in that configuration, there is no particular sequence to these things. Teeth show up when and where they show up.

If, however, one or more teeth do not appear after most of the others have come in, you might want to take your child to a dentist who specializes in child care. He or she may take an x-ray to check for impacted teeth (those stuck in the gums), and if such are found, dental surgery may need to be performed.

See TEETH in Appendix I: Norms and Values

Teeth Grinding

Known as *bruxism*, grinding of the teeth is usually done during sleep. It can severely damage the gums and supporting bone structures, eventually leading to a need for extensive periodontal work.

Sometimes children grind their teeth as a means of releasing tension caused by anxiety. Parents may notice a clenching of the teeth during the day and a tightening and relaxation of facial muscles as the child clenches and unclenches. At night the clenching may turn to grinding, often making enough noise to awaken parents. Frequently when the source of anxiety is identified and dealt with, the bruxism stops.

At other times teeth grinding can be an almost unconscious effort to relieve a poor bite when the jaws are closed. The child is attempting to create better contact by grinding away bad pressure spots.

In either instance, a dentist can fit the child with night guards, removable splints that fit over the tops of the teeth and correct the poor biting pressure. In order to prevent periodontal damage, these night guards should be worn whenever the child goes to bed. The child's doctor may also prescribe mild tranquilizers until the teeth-grinding habit is broken.

Teething

This is the normal eruption or cutting through the gums of a baby's first set of teeth, called the deciduous or milk teeth, and sometimes the "baby teeth."

There is extremely wide variation in the times at which teething occurs. A few babies are born with one or more front teeth; in other children, teeth may erupt as much as six or more months later than the overall average age. Parents should not consider either extreme abnormal. Nor should they use average teething times as a guide to their child's development; professionals do not use it as an index of growth and development, so why should parents?

In addition to using the table included in Appendix I: Norms and Values, another way of figuring out the average teething schedule is to take the child's age in months and subtract six. That is the *approximate* number of teeth.

Many babies seem to suffer no discomfort while teething. Others become very irritable, drool excessively, and communicate their discomfort by prolonged, almost incessant crying. They are often particularly restless at night, especially when the first four molars — the grinders — erupt.

Babies like to chew on almost anything, so parents can oblige their teething child with a clean washcloth, as the coarseness appears to be soothing, or a frequently washed teething ring, which should ideally not contain fluid, which could be contaminated. Parents may also gently massage the youngster's gums, which provides some direct relief from discomfort and also establishes the close parental contact fretful babies need.

If the baby continues to cry, becomes severely irritable, or shows any signs of fever, take the child to his or her doctor or health-care professional. Teething occurs at a time when an infant's antibody (infection-fighter) level is not at its peak yet, and what is perceived as teething may actually be an illness.

Temper Tantrum

Temper tantrums — flailing of the arms, lying on the floor and kicking, and loud screaming — tend to occur between the ages of two and four, especially during the infamous "terrible twos." Embarrassing as these spells may be to parents caught in the middle of a supermarket aisle or on a visit to grandparents, there are explanations for the behavior that may help parents better understand the child's position.

Youngsters of two to four are just beginning to develop a keen awareness of motor activity and how they can display their own prowess at moving about in extreme ways. This coincides with a time during which very few children are not experiencing verbal difficulties — they sense an inferiority at being unable to express themselves in clear language. Finally, few children of this young age group have managed to acquire any capacity for dealing with delayed gratification — they want what they want when they want it.

During the temper tantrum itself, attempts to intervene are almost hopeless. Communication is essentially impossible. If possible, parents should remove the child to a more suitable area until he or she finishes.

The temper tantrum should *never* gain children what they want, or a negative precedent will be set. Both parents should agree on what limits are set for their child, and disciplinary measures should be followed to the letter. Physical punishment only backfires to provoke increases in tantrum behavior. Punishment, which should be consistently followed, may consist of confining the child to a safe but solitary area of the house for a short time, temporarily depriving the child of a favorite book or toy, or whatever similar measures fit best with the particular family's life-style. The object is to deprive the child of his or her usual role in the ongoing activities of life in the household.

Although it may not be possible to avoid temper tantrums altogether, parents can do a lot to minimize or shorten them. It is especially important that parents not fly off the handle when something goes wrong. This clues the child that tantrums are an acceptable way to deal with anger or frustration. Parents should not expect too much of a toddler; he or she finds it almost unbearably frustrating to try to sit quietly while adults talk about adult subjects. Whenever appropriate, bring the child into a conversation. Avoiding unnecessary frustration can also help; children are far more prone to throw a temper tantrum when they are overfatigued or hungry.

Children should also be rewarded for good behavior. Verbal praise, a hug, a pat on the back, and smiles are important feedback for the child. Parents should make it clear to the child how well he or she has behaved and how good behavior is socially acceptable while bad behavior is not.

Usually the temper-tantrum stage passes within a few months. If it persists for a longer period of time, if it seems particularly violent and threatening, if it is indulged in by an older child, or if other signs of emotional disturbance are present, then parents should check with the child's doctor and possibly seek psychological counseling.

Compare BREATH HOLDING

Temperature, Taking of

Although fevers can become quite elevated (104° F and higher) before they endanger a child, it is important for parents to know a child's temperature if there seems to be something wrong or they suspect a particular illness. But how best to take the temperature?

Although many parents may not like it — and most children will not be thrilled either — the very best way to get an accurate reading is by taking the temperature rectally. Many doctors feel that axillary (armpit) temperatures are not very accurate and therefore not very valuable, and oral temperature taking may be difficult if not impossible in infants.

See FEVER

Terminal Illness in Children

Coming to terms with the approaching death of a child is certainly the most difficult task a parent must face. No matter how loving and supportive the family is, parents may derive more help from consulting with a professional who specializes in this area — a health-care professional, psychologist, social worker, specially trained members of the clergy, or a specialist in the subject of death and dying called a *thanatologist* — or meeting with a local chapter of one of the organizations formed by parents of fatally ill or deceased children.

Support is of tremendous help as parents try, daily, to lead as normal a life as is possible for the child, offering comfort during painful medical procedures, discussing whatever feelings and fears the child brings up, and trying to balance concern against undue attention that only adds to the child's own anxiety.

By the age of seven or eight, children can tell, from the behavior of those around them and from the likely need for frequent and lengthy hospitalizations, that something quite serious is going on. It was once thought that younger children did not have much concern about death and did not really understand its meaning. That may not be true; even preschool children have some idea of total disappearance, and the fear of going away forever may haunt young terminally ill children, as well as older children and adolescents. Parents who seek professional counseling for themselves are in a better position to deal with the fright and turmoil their fatally ill child may express verbally or behaviorally.

See also DEATH OF PARENT OR SIBLING

Throat Clearing

Nasal drainage that flows toward the back of the throat often causes children to make hacking or snarling noises in an effort to clear the fluid. Occasionally it results from obstructed air flow, as may be the case with enlarged tonsils and adenoids. The child should be taken to a doctor so the cause can be determined and treated. An ALLERGY or upper-respiratory infection may be at fault in producing chronic throat irritations and increased nasal secretions.

At times throat clearing becomes a habit, one that can become quite annoying. This seemingly minor situation can be difficult to cope with: Undue attention may increase the behavior because it gets attention, and ignoring it altogether may increase it in further efforts to gain attention. One approach is simply to explain to the child that the habit is extremely annoying. Suggest that whenever the urge to clear the throat is felt, the child substitute some acceptable and non-obtrusive behavior such as drinking a glass of water. If successful, offer the child praise for his or her willpower and grown-up behavior.

Thumb Sucking

The sucking response is one of an infant's earliest reflexes, present from the moment of birth. The nourishment taken in and the comfort associated with feeding become quickly translated into a means of soothing and relaxation associated with sucking itself. Parents can provide a pacifier to substitute for a thumb or fingers, but the response is the same: sucking.

Parental overconcern about a child's thumb sucking is quite often nothing more than making much ado about nothing. A child normally outgrows this behavior by about the age of five, frequently because playmates tease the child about baby behavior. Generally speaking, this normal rite of passage should be allowed; parents do not really need to interfere, and they should carefully avoid cajoling, teasing, or punishing a preschooler who continues to thumb suck. Neither should parents use severe measures such as painting the thumb with an obnoxious substance or making the child wear mittens. The puckered thumb, the old belief that thumb sucking interferes with language development, and the fear that thumb sucking will cause serious dental or gum problems before the eruption of permanent teeth are all concerns the parents can safely forget about.

Some parents, however, may wish to have a dentist fit the roof of the child's mouth with a training device that prevents the thumb from touching the roof of the mouth, thus discouraging thumb sucking. The real key, however, remains the child's own wish to stop this behavior, and, left to their own devices, most children do so at a time that is most appropriate for them. Of course, if the behavior persists well into the school years and/or is associated with EMOTIONAL WITHDRAWAL or other behavior problems, parents should seek psychological help.

See REGRESSIVE BEHAVIOR

Tooth Discoloration

Many factors can affect the color of teeth. Babies may sprout darkened teeth if the mother was given tetracycline during the second half of her pregnancy. This also occurs when children under the age of eight are given tetracycline.

Once a tooth has lost its nerve and blood-vessel supply — that is, when it is dead — it appears gray. Abnormal calcium metabolism, as in rickets, discolors children's teeth, as does high fever suffered during the time youngsters are forming tooth enamel. Excessive intake of fluoride can cause a mottling or discoloration of tooth enamel, but this should not happen if water-supply fluoridation does not exceed the recommended levels of one part fluoride per million parts of water.

Gross and permanent discoloration of the teeth can pose severe emotional problems for children. Parents may wish to consult with the child's dentist about the possibility of using techniques in which harmless enamel-colored material is applied for cosmetic purposes.

Tooth Loss

By the time children are about three years old, they should be checked by a dentist and begin various mouth-hygiene rituals. If a baby tooth is traumatically lost before the permanent teeth are coming in, parental first aid may help the dentist save the tooth.

If possible, stick the tooth back into its socket and hold it there or have the child hold it in position. Otherwise wrap the tooth in a wet towel or put it into a container of water so that vital tissues are not removed. Then take the child to the dentist *immediately* so that the tooth can be professionally replaced in its socket. Several procedures may be done, such as root canal work and wiring the tooth to secure it in place.

Tremors

From time to time, physiologic tremors — involuntary quivering of the muscles — may occur in otherwise healthy children; for example, they may begin to shake when they are intensely anxious.

Persistent tremors demand prompt medical evaluation because they may indicate an underlying disease or disorder, such as one that affects nerves or muscle groups.

Compare FEVER CONVULSIONS, SEIZURE DISORDERS

Type A Behavior

Type A people tend to be nervous, aggressive, and obsessed with details, exhibiting stress-related behavior patterns caused by a strong need to achieve and an equally strong desire for approval.

We tend to think of the typical Type A personality as some overworked businessman — always trying to shove 20 hours of work into an 8-hour day. Time is his enemy — there is not enough of it, and it is never utilized to his satisfaction. Type A behavior personalities — with their intense and sometimes hostile attitudes, their impatiently bouncing knees, their compulsion to acquire more and more, and their inability to waste time standing in lines ("hurry sickness") — are linked to coronary artery disease.

How does this relate to youngsters? There is no indication that there are legions of preteens roaring down the hallways of life, looking at their watches and teetering on the verge of heart attacks. But today there seem to be more and greater pressures on children to succeed, achieve, and excel than ever before. Their days are packed with school and after-school classes, extracurricular activities, and private lessons. They are trying to cram a lot of activity into a little time. And some youngsters are ill-prepared for such scheduling and demands. Some of them may already be displaying Type A behavior; others are being programmed to have it become a looming problem in later life.

Parents need to take a step back, look objectively at their well-intentioned desires to have their children be the best and the brightest, and determine whether the child is experiencing undue stress because of it or anxiety because he or she is not designed to handle such pressure well. Sometimes, mid-course corrections well before mid-life can be lifesavers.

U

Umbilical Cord

When the umbilical cord is cut at delivery, a small stump of it is left. Attending personnel generally paint it with a drying, antibacterial dye. It takes about a week to ten days before the cord stump falls off; in some cases, this may not occur for three or four weeks. When it falls off, small amounts of oozing and bleeding are normal.

During this healing time, parents should apply alcohol to the base of the cord at least twice a day or whenever the baby's diapers are changed. This dabbing with alcohol should be continued for several days after the cord falls off, then stopped when the area is clean and remains dry.

If there is no sign of infection (such as unusual drainage), nothing more need be done. Large amounts of thick yellow-colored material, especially if foul smelling, may indicate a bacterial infection. Redness spreading away from the base of the cord and onto the skin of the abdominal wall signals a spread of infection. Since newborns cannot localize infections very well — that is, infections tend to spread from one location over larger areas — medical evaluation is needed to see whether antibiotics are required.

Sometimes after the cord has fallen off, a small red elevation — called an *umbilical granuloma* — remains on the cord stump, representing an area that has not healed completely, and yellow-red drainage may occur. Cauterization performed by a doctor usually allows for rapid healing. In extremely rare circumstances, there may be an abnormal connection between the base of the cord and another structure within the abdominal cavity. As a result of this abnormality, large amounts of clear urine-like fluid may drain from the cord stump. Newborns with this condition should be taken to a doctor as soon as possible.

Underachievement

Parents should be realistic about children's underachievement — the failure to perform at a level consistent with his or her abilities. It is natural for parents to think that their children are brighter, more creative, more talented, and more motivated than they are. A professor of literature may be baffled when her small daughter shows no more than an average aptitude for talking, reading, and writing. A master mechanic may be dumbfounded when his six-year-old son shows no interest in building a small engine.

When parents are quite sure they have not overestimated their child's abilities — and objective assessment by a professional is the best way to be sure — then they should look for environmental stresses. The true underachiever is usually angry and frustrated, often because he or she senses an inability to measure up to what is expected. A classic example is that of teachers who overpraise an older sibling, so that the younger child feels inadequate as a student, even when he or she is intrinsically just as bright as the older brother or sister. It is important for the parents and other adults to stop applying undue pressure and begin to praise and reward a child for what he or she *does* do well.

If the problem continues and/or worsens, a medical evaluation is necessary to make sure there is no slowly developing chronic illness or no vision or hearing problem that may be interfering with the child's performance. DEPRESSION also lowers the child's urge to excel, or even to perform at all.

Underweight

Children who are thin are not necessarily ill. During the growing years, a child's weight becomes important only if there is a consistent failure to gain weight or a significant loss of weight.

If the child's level of activity and increase in height are normal, the thin child faces fewer problems with weight control as an adult. Weight-to-height proportions should be kept in mind, especially within the framework of the genetic characteristics the child may reasonably be expected to have. However, slavishly following charts of average weight gains anticipated for certain age groups may cause more parental concern than is warranted.

It is extremely unusual for a child to lose weight while growing.

The evidence should be documented by at least a couple of weight measurements or, if a child levels off and gains no more weight over a period of several weeks, a doctor should examine the child. Infants may fail to gain if they have PYLORIC STENOSIS or chronic diarrhea; adolescents, especially girls, may lose weight with ANOREXIA NERVOSA. Signs and symptoms besides weight loss from these conditions generally cause parents to seek medical help.

Urine and Urination

The amount and the color of a child's urine are directly related to the amount and the types of fluids and foods taken in. When they are active, thirsty children take in large amounts of fluids and void a large volume of urine that is very light colored because there is more water than waste products. When less fluids are drunk and a larger amount of waste substances must be removed from the body, this concentration of material results in a dark-colored urine.

Variations in color, ranging from barely yellowish through straw color to amber, are common and normal. Appearance varies too. At times, urine looks cloudy because normal crystals are present. If the urine is allowed to cool and sit, the cloudiness increases.

Children's control over urination comes a little later than their control over bowel movements. Daytime control is usually achieved by the age of three or four years; BED-WETTING and daytime accidents generally stop by about age five.

Parents generally need not concern themselves about the frequency and appearance of their children's urine unless other symptoms and signs are present. For example, greater frequency and dilute urine may suggest DIABETES MELLITUS if accompanied by unusually excessive thirst. Painful and frequent urination, BLOOD IN THE URINE, and AB-DOMINAL PAIN could signal CYSTITIS. A KIDNEY INFECTION OR DISEASE is likely when these same signs and symptoms are also accompanied by fever or vomiting. An acute inflammation of the kidneys may be present if, in addition to frequent voiding, the urine is obviously bloody or the color of very dark tea. Bloody urine after an injury indicates damage somewhere along the urinary tract. All these symptoms require medical attention.

V

Vegetarianism

Whether it be for health reasons — to cut down on saturated fats and cholesterol because of fears of heart disease and other ailments — or for ethical reasons brought about by animal-rights attitudes, more and more Americans are considering a meatless diet. But there has been a concern that children cannot thrive as vegetarians because they will not get the vitamins, proteins, and other nutrients required for continued health and growth.

This is not the case. There is no reason why anyone — child or adult — cannot survive well on a vegetarian regimen. In fact, studies of other societies and groups, such as the non-meat-eating Seventh Day Adventists, indicate that a vegetarian diet — whether ovo-lacto (eggs and milk products permitted) or vegan (no animal products whatever) — can be extremely healthful and even weight reducing, and should not stunt the growth of youngsters. Certainly, care must be taken to assure that meals include items that provide enough protein in addition to vitamins A, B_2, B_{12}, and D, as well as certain minerals and amino acids. And despite long-held views to the contrary, little or no extra time is required to devise and prepare a vegetarian meal instead of a conventional, meat-centered one.

It might not be wise to attempt to provide a balanced vegetarian diet for youngsters without dairy products being available. They need the calcium and other minerals and vitamins that milk and cheeses provide. Low-fat and nonfat forms of popular dairy products are readily available in most markets, and these afford children the nutritional benefits without the fat and cholesterol drawbacks. Just to be on the safe side, children on vegan diets should be given vitamin and mineral supplements, especially for B_{12} and iron.

Doctors, many of whom are not well-versed in the ways of diet and nutrition, may provide charts of foodstuffs and their vitamin and mineral contents, along with other information — and possibly a caution about the dangers of vegetarianism, which they may only vaguely understand. If your doctor or health-care professional is not very helpful or is even discouraging, and going meatless is your desire, then there are many books, pamphlets, and recipe sources that can help you. Also, check with nutritionists or even health-food stores about vegetarian groups or organizations in your area.

Voice Change

In adolescence, the voices of both boys and girls change into those of men and women as the larynx (voice box) enlarges and the vocal cords assume adult size, alignment, and tautness.

Customarily, however, people tend to think in terms of the male voice change because of the more pronounced difference, which is caused by gender differences in voice-box and vocal-cord structuring. Cracking and sudden slides from deep bass to high soprano are normal in male adolescents. Parents, as well as siblings and other adults, would do well to ignore these occurrences. The boy should never be teased or imitated, since this could inhibit his speaking and increase adolescent shyness.

See also HOARSENESS, LARYNGITIS

Vomiting

Vomiting in and of itself is not dangerous, except when a child is semiconscious or unconscious, in which case vomited material may seep back down into the lungs. It may accompany minor ailments and upsets that affect the stomach and intestines.

The greatest danger lies in the possibility of dehydration, a condition in which there is too much loss of body fluids and a salt imbalance occurs. The length of time before dehydration sets in varies. If either the frequency of urination or level of activity is decreased significantly, the child should see a doctor.

A good method for evaluating the possibility of danger is to follow these steps:

1. Give the child nothing to eat and drink for a period of one hour after he or she last vomits.
2. Then give the child one ounce of water.
3. Twenty minutes later give two ounces of water.

4. Twenty minutes later give three ounces of water.
5. If the child retains the water, proceed with other liquids and watch the level of activity and for urination. If the child vomits during this two-hour interval, call the doctor right away.

Young babies up to about one year can be given one of the balanced electrolyte solutions available in drug stores. These provide all the salts in appropriate concentrations for the vomiting infant. After a day or two, the regular formula can be used and those solid foods formerly eaten can be gradually reintroduced.

When the vomiting is over, older babies, as well as children and adolescents, can benefit from drinking heavily diluted syrup drinks, flattened ginger ale or cola, beef or chicken broth, and munching on crushed ice chips or popsicles. Milk and solid foods should be avoided for at least 24 hours, after which time the child can gradually resume a normal diet after starting with refined cereals, cookies, and applesauce but keeping away from raw vegetables for a few days.

Although it is true that vomiting is not serious or dangerous, it may indicate the presence of an infection or some other disease. Parents should remember that it is the combination of symptoms that is important. A pain in the right side of the abdomen with vomiting may mean APPENDICITIS. Vomiting and a stiff neck may mean MENINGITIS. Vomiting may also occur after sharp blows to the head.

Unless parents are reasonably sure that the vomiting is associated with nothing more than stomach upset from overeating, overexertion, or, say, a mild case of INFLUENZA, they should check with the child's doctor about the advisability of a physical examination. This precaution is especially important whenever there is blood in the vomitus or if accidental POISONING is suspected.

See also ABDOMINAL PAIN, COLIC, CYSTIC FIBROSIS, GASTROENTERITIS, HERNIA, INTESTINAL OBSTRUCTION, MILK ALLERGY

Weight Gain

After the spurt of growth in infancy and before the spurt common to adolescence, a child may generally be expected to gain approximately seven to ten pounds each year, accounting for the increased size of organs, bones, and other tissues.

The best way of assessing whether children are gaining too much weight is simply by looking at them and carefully seeing if they seem to fit their frames. Obesity in children is rarely the result of some glandular or hormonal problem. There is a strong hereditary influence, but the genetic factor may be overshadowed by the family's eating patterns. If more calories are taken in than are used by life functions and other body activities, the child becomes overweight. If a child becomes overweight during early childhood and remains so by the age of 11, the individual is at high risk of being obese for the rest of his or her life.

Treatment is aimed at altering caloric intake while increasing level of activity. Snacks should be eliminated except for raw fruits and vegetables, fruit-juice popsicles, and perhaps some sugarless gum to curb the appetite. Fluid intake should include at least six glasses of water a day; this can be supplemented by skim milk and unsweetened diet-type drinks. Meals should contain lots of protein in the form of cheese, eggs, and meats, and average portions should be served, with no seconds. Desserts are best confined to diet gelatins or fresh fruits.

Diets that cause very rapid weight loss are not advised. Neither should children be given appetite-reducing medications. A physician's or health-care professional's evaluation is recommended, and working with a dietician may further stimulate the child's desire to lose weight. Hand-drawn and colored reminders can be posted at particularly crucial spots such as the refrigerator door. The support of self-help groups — for example, summer camps where youngsters go to lose weight, or organizations at which overweight children can freely discuss their problems and successes — have proved valuable in many cases.

Parents, especially, need to cooperate by simply not having high-calorie foods, rich desserts, junk-food fillers, and nondiet soft drinks in the house.

X

X-Rays, Risks of

Radiation is, for all concerned parents, the good, the bad, and the scary. So many diagnostic explorations begin or end with x-rays, and so many illnesses and conditions are discovered through the use of ionizing radiation. Yet parents read so much about the dangers of exposing their children to radiation of all sorts. How do the risks and benefits stack up against each other?

One thing is certain: X-rays can cause cancers, and the young are as susceptible — even, it appears, *more* susceptible — than adults. X-rays of an infant can cause chromosomal damage resulting in cancer that shows up 20 or more years later; screening tests using x-rays, such as those for SCOLIOSIS, may expose children to a significant amount of radiation. Overdiagnosis, misdiagnosis, and overtesting can endanger children too.

On the other hand, much of this testing and screening is necessary, as are many dental x-rays. Until better, safer ways to get pictures of certain inner body areas are invented, x-rays will still be used, and rightly so, if they are properly, judiciously, and carefully ordered and executed.

Parents concerned about the effect of x-rays on their children need to act as consumer watchdogs on behalf of their children. They need to:

- Question doctors and other health-care professionals about the need for recommended x-rays, and always get second opinions about them.
- Ask if there are alternative imaging techniques that expose the child to less or no ionizing radiation.
- Be satisfied that the person doing the x-raying is qualified to do so; ask about the doctor's, dentist's, or technician's training and credentials.

• Know if the x-ray machinery is functioning properly, so that it does not give an excessive dose of radiation. Ask to see when the machine was last inspected by the appropriate state agency that checks such technical apparatus.

Do not be intimidated by professionals who may make you feel as if you are being a worrywart. If a doctor or health-care professional will not take you seriously in this regard, perhaps you should take your business elsewhere. After all, your child's future is at stake.

But as frightening as the prospect of your child being x-rayed may be, sometimes it is necessary. Sometimes it is the best or only way to see potential dangers inside your child. At these times, the possibility of radiation hazards has to be weighed against the certainty of finding a treatment or cure.

YOUR CHILD'S HEALTH RECORDS

Child's Name:

Length at Birth:

Weight at Birth:

Birthdate:

Hospital:

Formula:

GROWTH CHART

Age	Height	Weight

IMMUNIZATIONS

Immunization	Date	Comments
DPT/oral polio/Hib		
DPT/oral polio/Hib		

DPT/oral polio _____

Measles/Mumps/Rubella (MMR) _____

DPT/polio booster _____

DPT/polio booster _____

DT (tetanus toxoid and reduced diphtheria) _____

Tetanus booster _____

Tetanus booster _____

Allergies

Allergic Reactions to Medications:

PRESCRIPTIONS

Date	Number	Doctor	Prescribed for

ILLNESS AND INJURIES

Date

Problem

Treatment

HOSPITALIZATIONS

Date

Reason

Treatment

EMERGENCY MEDICAL CARE

Date

Reason

Treatment

DENTAL RECORDS

Date	Reason for Visit	Results

Pediatrician: _____
(name)
_____
(address)
_____
(telephone)

Dentist: _____
(name)
_____
(address)
_____
(telephone)

Norms and Values

The entries in this section should act as a general guide and early-warning system for parents curious or concerned about their children's mechanisms of life and health. Many of the numbers here are *ranges* or *approximations*, not hard-and-fast figures that must be met precisely. Everyone is an individual, and readings may vary.

Some of the statistics and values found in this section may also be found in entries throughout the book, but are collected here for fast and easy references.

Apgar Score

A minute after birth and then five minutes later, the baby is examined and given a rating of between 0 and 2 on five different health factors: color, muscle tone, heart rate, respiratory effort, and reflex irritability. The highest score is a 10 (2 points for each factor).

The Apgar scoring is used to predict the chances of survival and probability of health difficulties faced by a newborn. Children given Apgar scores of 2 have almost overwhelming odds against long-term survival, while those with 8 or more will almost certainly survive the neonatal phase.

Blood

The condition of the blood is demonstrated by testing for normal values established by checking large numbers of healthy individuals over a long period of time; the volume of red blood cells is measured by the hematocrit, while the oxygen-carrying capacity is measured by the hemoglobin percent. These normal values change according to the age of the child. For example, at birth an infant may show a hematocrit of between 48 and 50 percent and a hemoglobin of around 16 to 18 grams per 100 cubic centimeters (cc). Because red cell production normally falls off right after birth, both these measurements will fall to their lowest points between the first 8 to 12 weeks of life (approximately 35 percent and 11 to 12 grams per 100 cc, respectively). This falloff is normal and requires no therapy. Later on, children usually show a certain range that averages out to the following:

Age	Hematocrit, percent	Hemoglobin, percent
6 months–6 years	37	12
7 years–12 years	38	13
Over 12 years		
Females	42	14
Males	47	16

Blood Pressure

Blood pressure tends to vary according to a person's body position, level of activity, and other factors, but a school-age child's systolic (the top reading that measures the pressure of the heart at work during a beat) and diastolic (the bottom reading that measures the pressure of the heart at rest between beats) blood pressure measurements should probably never exceed $^{100}/_{80}$ (referred to as 100 over 80) or $^{110}/_{80}$.

Up to and including about the age of four, an average reading is $^{85}/_{60}$. Then, for a while, the top figure increases approximately 5 points with every 2 years of age added.

Age (years)	Blood Pressure
6	90/60
8	95/62
10	100/65

The increase then slows until the adolescent is about sixteen and should not exceed $^{118}/_{75}$.

See HYPERTENSION, HYPOTENSION

Breathing Rate

As an exchange of oxygen and carbon dioxide takes place in the lungs, adults breathe in and out approximately 16 times each minute. The breathing rate of children is typically higher than that of adults. This rate varies, depending on the child's physical activity, state of wakefulness or sleepiness, comfort or discomfort, and various emotional factors.

As a general guide for parents who may be interested, children's rates tend to follow these ranges:

Age	Expected Range (breaths per minute)
Newborns	30–40
Infants	20–30
1-year–adulthood	20

Parents should note that these figures are for expected *ranges*; the actual rate may vary from minute to minute. If your child's breathing rate is *consistently* over 40 per minute, there may be some heart or lung problem, and medical consultation is recommended.

Fitness

Although there are many indicators of physical fitness, including weight, blood pressure, and heart rate, among others, certain levels of physical attainment have been devised to gauge how fit a child really is. It is not recommended that you go out to a field with stopwatch and clipboard like a drill instructor and put your child through the rigors in order to satisfy yourself that he or she is physically fit. But in the course of play, in a casual, recreational manner, you might want to find out. However, do not impose these activities on children of questionable fitness until a physician has determined that you will not be endangering them by doing so.

	ONE-MILE RUN-WALK	
Age (years)	Boys	Girls
6	12 min., 36 sec.	13 min., 12 sec.
9	10 min., 30 sec.	11 min., 52 sec.
12	8 min., 40 sec.	11 min., 5 sec.

SIT-UPS		
Age (*years*)	Boys	Girls
6	22 per minute	23 per minute
12	40 per minute	35 per minute

HANGING FROM PULL-UP BAR		
Age (*years*)	Boys	Girls
6	At least 6 seconds	At least 5 seconds
12	At least 12 seconds	At least 7 seconds

Heart Rate

The hearts of infants and children beat much faster than the average 70 times a minute that is normal for adults.

Newborn babies have an average heart rate of 120 to 140; during bouts of crying or excessive activity, this may increase to 170 or more, whereas in sleep it drops to between 70 and 90.

As the child grows older, the rate slows. By 4 to 6 years of age, the heart rate is about 100 beats per minute; by the age of 8 to 10, it drops to an average of 90. It reaches adult level by late adolescence.

Parents should keep in mind that these are *averages*. For example, a 6-year-old may have a heart rate as low as 75 or as high as 115 and still be within the normal range. Also, from about age 12 to 18, girls' heart rates tend to be approximately 5 points higher than boys'.

Just as in adults, children's heart rates are affected by strenuous activity, excitement, fear, and various other emotional states, as well as by certain drugs, foods, and drinks such as excessive coffee and cigarettes. It is only when children over 8 or 10 years old consistently show a heart rate of 120 or more that parents should arrange for a medical examination to determine whether there is some serious underlying cause for the fast beating.

Motor Development

There is a great deal of variation within the age ranges at which children develop certain motor skills—that is, the capacity to perform certain movements and tasks. Nonetheless, some general expectations may be helpful to parents, but they should not worry unduly if their child seems to fall behind other children slightly.

Age	Activity
Birth	Grasp reflex (able to hold parent's finger)
3–4 months	Sits if supported
4–5 months	Can reach intentionally
7–8 months	Sits alone
6–10 months	Grasps with palm, grasps with thumb and forefinger
12–13 months	Stands alone briefly
12–15 months	Walks briefly without assistance
2 years	Climbs on furniture, walks up stairs one at a time, can build six-block tower
3 years	Can ride tricycle, build three-block bridge, make a cross with a crayon
3–6 years	Adds many more skills, such as skating or jumping rope, as muscles strengthen and speed increases
7 years	Can bathe self, use a crayon to copy a drawing of a diamond, tie a bow knot
8 years	Can use table knife
9 years	Bathes without assistance

Speech

Despite the wide variations in the time a child begins to speak, parents can use the following information as a rough guide to what can usually be expected.

Age	Vocalizations
3–5 weeks	Throaty noises of an indistinct, almost primitive nature
10–12 weeks	Cooing sounds, often in response to adult speech
3–6 months	Babbling is added to the cooing; this may lead to forming the words "mama" or "dada," and the child may even point to the individual
10–12 months	Single words, for example, "cat," "dog," "milk"
2 years	Two-word phrases
3 years	Three-word sentences, for example, "I want milk."
4 years	Six- or seven-word sentences, for example, "I want milk with chocolate, please."

Teeth

Most parents are interested in having some guide to teething expectations. The following table is included with the reminder that it is only a rough guide.

Age (*months*)	Teeth
5–9	Two lower front teeth
8–12	Four upper front teeth
12–15	Two lower (side) front teeth
10–16	Four first molars (upper and lower)
16–20	Four canines (third teeth from center, upper and lower)
20–30	Four second molars (upper and lower, the so-called second-year molars)

Temperature

Ranges for normal body temperatures are:

Rectal	98°–100°F	36.6°–37.8°C
Oral	97°–99°F	36.1°–37.1°C
Axillary (armpit)	98°–98°F	35.6°–37.8°C

Physicians, Practitioners, and Specialists

The following is a list of health-care professionals that may at one time or another be called in to care for your child. Each is followed by a brief description of what they specialize in and what they are empowered to do. Keep in mind that a license to practice medicine is not a restrictive license; that is, once a person has a medical license, he or she can practice any branch of medicine he or she wants to. That is why it is always safer to use board-certified specialists—those who have had extra and continual training and have passed exams in their areas of specialization.

Allergist — Specializes in diagnosis and treatment of allergic conditions such as ASTHMA, HAY FEVER, and skin sensitivities.

Anesthesiologist — Specialist medical doctor who dispenses anesthetics and monitors the safety of the patient under anesthesia during operations.

Cardiologist — A medical heart specialist.

Dentist — General practitioner in the care and treatment of teeth, gums, and surrounding bone structure.

Dermatologist — Specializes in diseases of the skin.

Emergency Medicine — The specialty of emergency-room medicine.

Endocrinologist — Specializing in the treatment of diseases and disorders of the endocrine system, which includes the pituitary and thyroid glands, as well as the pancreas and its diabetic problems.

Family Medicine — Specializes in office-based, full-spectrum care; differs from a general practitioner in amount of extra education.

Gastroenterologist — Specializes in treating disorders of the gastrointestinal tract.

General Practitioner — Nonspecialist physician with office-oriented, first-line-of-defense practice.

Gynecologist — Specializes in examining and treating diseases of the female reproductive system.

Hematologist — Specializes in diagnosing and treating diseases of the blood and blood system.

Immunologist — Specializes in disorders involving the body's immune system, such as AIDS and autoimmune diseases.

Internist — Specializes in diagnosis and treatment, nonsurgically, of diseases; frequently in family practice, often in a specific subspecialty.

Licensed Practical Nurse — Licensed caregiver with vocational training in nursing; training and education is usually less thorough than that of a registered nurse.

Nephrologist — Specializes in diagnosing and treating diseases of the kidney.

Neurologist — Examines, diagnoses, and cares for diseases of the nervous system.

Neurosurgeon — Specializes in alleviating problems of the brain, nerves, and spinal cord through surgery.

Nurse Practitioner — A registered nurse who has gone on to acquire further medical education, permitting him or her to practice a broad but limited level of diagnosis and treatment; nurse practitioners often work with or in place of doctors in office, hospital, or health maintenance organization (HMO) settings.

Oncologist — Diagnoses and treats cancerous conditions.

Ophthalmologist — Medical doctor who examines, diagnoses, and may perform surgery to treat diseases of and injuries to the eye. Not to be confused with an *optometrist*, a nonmedical practitioner who examines the eye in order to prescribe corrective lenses.

Orthopedist — Often subspecializing in surgical approaches, this doctor deals with problems involving the musculoskeletal system.

Osteopathic Physician — A doctor of osteopathic medicine (D.O.) who has taken a full course of medical training in most ways identical to those of an allopathic medical doctor (M.D.), but in addition has learned manipulative therapy in which the musculoskeletal and spinal areas are repositioned as a therapeutic mode.

Otorhinolaryngologist — Specializes in treating illness and disease in the ear, nose, and throat. Often referred to as an ENT specialist, and someone frequently seen by ear-infected children.

Pediatrician — Specializes in diseases and conditions affecting humans from infancy until adolescence.

Physician Assistant — Similar in many ways to nurse practitioners, this paraprofessional carries out many of the functions of a physician, but works under a physician's supervision.

Plastic Surgeon — Rebuilds parts of the body damaged by accident or disease, or to correct congenital (present-at-birth) or growth-induced structural malformations. This professional also performs so-called cosmetic surgery, used to make faces and bodies seem prettier and conform with current societal standards.

Podiatrist — Specializes in diagnosing and treating diseases and conditions of the feet.

Proctologist — Examines and treats diseases of the colon, rectum, and anus.

Psychiatrist — Medical doctor specializing in the care and prevention of mental illness through the use of psychoanalysis, medication, or, if necessary, referral to a neurosurgeon.

Radiologist — Medical doctor who studies radiation-produced images, such as x-ray pictures, to aid in the diagnosis and treatment of disease.

Registered Nurse — Licensed caregiver with high degree of training and skills; RNs usually have received at least two extra years of education beyond that of licensed practical nurses, and may have received their nursing degrees as part of a broader college education program.

Thoracic Surgeon — Operates on structures within the chest area, including the heart, lungs, and esophagus.

Urologist — Diagnoses and treats diseases of the urinary system.

APPENDIX III

Directory of Poison-Control Information Telephone Numbers

By calling the following numbers, organized alphabetically by state, you can get help and information about procedures and antidotes in case poison is ingested by your child. Some of these numbers are direct-dial help lines, while others are the extensions for the state's health department or emergency-services division.

To be prepared for an emergency poisoning situation, call the number for your state to make certain you have the emergency number for your locality as well as the procedures to follow in case of a poisoning. You may also be able to find your locality's poison-control phone number at the front of your telephone directory, or in the blue pages listing government agencies in your regular phone book.

Write down the emergency poison-control telephone number for your area (as well as the direct extension number for the nearest hospital emergency room and, perhaps, the number of your community ambulance service) in the appropriate space provided at the front of this book, as well as in several spots in your house immediately adjacent to and easily reached from telephones, such as on a bulletin board, on the refrigerator, on a nightstand, and so on. If your telephone has one-touch or memory dialing, enter the emergency number for fast access.

Be prepared—do not wait for an emergency and then have to frantically search for the phone number. Have it handy.

Finally, in an extreme emergency, you can always call the police or fire emergency number, which in most areas is 911.

Alabama — 1-800-462-0800 or 205-292-6678

Alaska — 907-261-3193

Arizona — 1-800-362-0101

Arkansas — 501-661-6161

California — 916-445-4171

Colorado — 303-331-8630

Connecticut — 203-566-4800 or 203-566-7336

Delaware — 302-655-3389

District of Columbia — 202-625-3333

Florida — 904-487-1566

Georgia — 1-800-282-5846

Hawaii — 808-735-5267

Idaho — 1-800-632-8000

Illinois — 1-800-942-5969 or 217-782-4977

Indiana — 1-800-382-9097

Iowa — 1-800-362-2327

Kansas — 913-296-1500

Kentucky — 502-564-3970

Louisiana — 504-342-4881

Maine — 1-800-442-6305

Maryland — 1-800-492-2414 (in Baltimore: 301-528-7701)

Massachusetts — 617-232-2120

Michigan — 1-800-632-2727 or 1-800-462-6642

Minnesota — 612-347-3141

Mississippi — 601-987-3880

Missouri — 314-751-6400

Montana — 1-800-525-5042

Nebraska — 1-800-955-9119

Nevada — 702-687-3065

New Hampshire — 1-800-562-8236

New Jersey — 1-800-962-1253

New Mexico — 505-843-2551

New York — 518-474-2121

North Carolina — 1-800-672-1697

North Dakota — 1-800-732-2200 (in Bismarck: 701-223-4357)

Ohio — 614-466-3543

Oklahoma — 1-800-522-4611 or 405-271-5454

Oregon — 503-229-5586

Pennsylvania — 1-800-692-7254
Rhode Island — 401-277-5727
South Carolina — 803-734-5000
South Dakota — 1-800-952-0123
Tennessee — 615-367-6278
Texas — 409-765-1420 or 512-458-7111
Utah — 801-538-6435
Vermont — 802-658-3456
Virginia — 1-800-523-6019
Washington — 1-800-525-0127
West Virginia — 1-800-642-3625 or 304-348-3956
Wisconsin — 608-266-1511
Wyoming — 1-800-442-2702 (in Cheyenne: 307-635-9256)

APPENDIX IV

Additional Toll-Free Numbers

In addition to the toll-free numbers for information, treatment, and support-group referrals that appear in the appropriate entries elsewhere in this volume, there are some other more general services available. These are briefly listed here. Should these numbers be changed before this book's publication date, or if you believe that a group offering information and aid concerning a disease or condition has a toll-free number, call the 800 number directory-assistance operator at 800-555-1212.

American Medical Association American Medical Radio News 800-448-9384 (latest medical news)

American Mental Health Fund — 800-433-5959

American Osteopathic Association — 800-621-1773

Beech-Nut Nutrition Hot Line — 800-523-6633, 9 A.M. to 5 P.M. eastern time

Chemical Referral Center of the Chemical Manufacturers Association — 800-CMA-8200, 9 A.M. to 6 P.M. eastern time (information on household chemicals)

Child Abuse Hot Line — 800-422-4453

Child Care Information Service — 800-424-2460 (information on child-care services)

Children's Hospital International — 800-24-CHILD (information and referral on hospice services)

Consumer Product Safety Commission — 800-638-CPSC

Environmental Protection Agency National Pesticide Information Clearinghouse — 800-858-7378 (806-743-3091 in Texas)

Gerber Products Company — 800-443-7237

Medic Alert Foundation — 800-ID-ALERT (for medical-condition ID bracelets)

National Information Center for Orphan Drugs and Rare Diseases — 800-456-3505

National Library of Medicine — 800-272-4787 or 800-638-8480

National Pesticide Telecommunications Network — 800-858-7378

National Second Opinion Surgical Program of the Department of Health and Human Services — 800-638-6833 (800-492-6603 in Maryland)

Office of Disease Prevention and Health Promotion of the National Health Information Center — 800-336-4797

Parents Without Partners — 800-637-7974 (301-588-9356 in Maryland)

Shriner's Hospital Referral Line — 800-237-5055, 8 A.M. to 5 P.M. eastern time (800-282-9161 in Florida) (information on services at Shriner's Hospital)

Vitamin Hot Line — 800-533-VITA

Youth With Disabilities — 800-333-6293

Glossary

acute — having symptoms that are painful or severe, but last only a short length of time.

allergen — substance that causes an allergic reaction.

alveoli — the small air passages in the lungs.

amino acid — one of the elements that form proteins; fifteen of them can be produced by the body, while the other ten must be made available to the body in the form of food.

amniocentesis — surgical procedure in which a small amount of fluid from the amniotic sac (which encloses the fetus) is removed in order to examine it for signs of possible defects in the unborn child.

androgenic — having to do with the hormone that produces male characteristics in a child.

antibiotic — a chemical substance produced by certain species of bacteria, molds, or other microorganisms that can kill other species of germs or inhibit their growth and multiplication. Antibiotics are among the very few drugs that can cure a disease by removing its cause. Penicillin was one of the first of the modern antibiotics to be discovered.

antibodies — a protein molecule that attacks substances the body reacts negatively to; a "soldier" in the immune system's defense network.

arrhythmia — abnormal rhythm or disturbance of the heartbeat.

bradycardia — abnormally slow heartbeat.

311

breech birth — situation in which the fetus emerges from the birth canal backwards; that is, instead of headfirst, it presents with its buttocks or feet first.

bruise — medically known as a *contusion*, this is a tissue injury caused by a sudden impact or crushing injury. The skin remains unbroken, but discoloration results from the rupturing of tiny blood vessels.

bruxism — the act of grinding one's teeth while asleep.

carbohydrate — made up of carbon, hydrogen, and oxygen, it is a ready source of energy from food.

CAT scan — a method of getting images of the interior parts of the body in pictures that are essentially layers, or slices, of the organ or structure imaged.

chromosome — a structure in animal cells that contains DNA (deoxyribonucleic acid), the determinant of genetic information and heredity.

chronic — description of a condition that lasts a long time, showing little or no improvement or change. *See* ACUTE.

cyst — a small sac, usually containing some sort of fluid or other substance.

dehydration — the bodily state caused by having lost or received insufficient amounts of water.

dermatitis — skin inflammation.

diaphragm — the horizontal muscular wall that separates the chest cavity from the abdominal region.

diarrhea — excessively loose and frequent bowel movements.

diastolic — the lower measure of blood pressure that measures the pressure of the heart at rest between beats.

edema — an abnormal accumulation of fluid resulting in swelling.

electrocardiogram (EKG) — a graphic depiction of electrical activity in the heart. It is made on a machine called an electrocardiograph.

electroencephalogram (EEG) — a graphic depiction of electrical activity in the brain. It is made on a machine called an electroencephalograph.

endocrine — having to do with glands that secrete hormones.

enuresis — the medical term for bed-wetting.

fontanel — the so-called soft spot on an infant's head where the skull has not completely closed up.

gamma globulin — a substance composed of antibodies and used to help in the fight against a massive infection.

histamine — a normal body substance concentrated largely in those tissues that have direct or indirect contact with the air and that, in the case of injury or infection, is released into affected tissues because it causes a dilation, or opening, of the smaller blood vessels at the site of an injury and contributes to the so-called inflammatory response, which is a natural feature of the healing process.

hypoallergenic — descriptive of a substance that is less likely to cause an allergic reaction than other substances of the same type.

hypothalamus — a part of the brain that controls many important bodily functions.

incubator — a device that is heated and maintains a controlled environment for newborn premature babies.

infection — state or condition in which organs or tissues are invaded by pathogenic (disease-causing) organisms.

IQ — short for intelligence quotient, it is a measure of a human's intelligence.

larynx — commonly known as the voice box, it is the structure in human throats that contains the vocal cords.

leukocyte — white blood cells that help in the fight against infections.

malignant — descriptive of a cancer that is not under control, will become worse, and will probably lead to death. The opposite of this is *benign*.

meconium — dark green substance in fetuses' intestines that becomes the material of their first bowel movements.

menarche — the onset of menstruation.

metastasis — descriptive of a cancer that is spreading throughout the body.

molding — the head of the baby being forced into the shape of the birth canal during delivery.

mucous membranes — the lining of the tubular organs of the body.

periodontal — having to do with the gums and other tissues holding the teeth in place.

peritoneum — the thin, smooth, almost transparent, moist membrane that lines the walls of the abdominal cavity and parts of internal organs.

plasma — the fluid part of the blood, not including the red and white blood cells.

platelet — a flat, disc-shaped component of the blood that tends to stick onto damaged surfaces and is responsible for the clotting of blood.

polyp — a mass that grows out from a mucous membrane; sometimes they are considered tumors. Though usually benign, they can be malignant.

psychoactive — affecting behavior and the workings of the mind.

puberty — the time of life when secondary sex characteristics (development of breasts, onset of menstruation in girls; appearance of facial hair and voice changes in boys) start to develop; it is also the time when sexual reproduction becomes possible.

retina — a lining inside the eye, at the back, that contains photoreceptors connected to the brain by the optic nerve.

sebaceous glands — glands that secrete sebum—a colorless, odorless, oily substance—onto the skin by way of the hair follicles.

sigmoidoscope — a diagnostic tool used for direct observation and examination of the colon.

spinal tap — a procedure in which some of the cerebrospinal fluid is removed from the spine for diagnostic purposes.

syncope — fainting.

systolic — the upper measure of blood pressure that measures the pressure of the heart at work during a beat.

tachycardia — abnormally fast heart rate.

tetracycline — a commonly prescribed antibiotic that is effective against a wide array of microorganisms.

tourniquet — a device—usually a cloth or something that is flexible and can be folded or tied—used to stem the flow of blood to a point farther away from the heart.

tracheotomy — a surgical incision through the neck into the trachea, or windpipe.

tumor — a growth of tissue, either benign or malignant, that is aggressive in its growth. Sometimes referred to as a *neoplasm*.

ultrasound — descriptive of a technique in which parts deep within the body can be imaged by recording the echoes of ultrasonic waves aimed at those parts.

upper-respiratory infection — an inflammation of structures in the nose and throat areas caused by viral or bacterial infection.

urethra — the tube through which urine passes from the bladder out of the body.

INDEXES

Index by Region of Body Affected

Mental/Emotional

Stomach/Midsection

Other/Nonspecific

Symptom Index

Note: Entries without page numbers are cross-references to this index.

Abdomen. See Stomach.

Achiness. See Influenza, 93–94; Lyme disease, 103–4; Rabies, 129; Rubella 135–36

behind eyes. See Sinusitis, 144–45

Appetite, changes in, 175–76. See also Addiction, warning signs of, 173–74

increase in. See Appetite, changes in, 175–76; Tapeworms, 154

weight loss and. See Thyroid disorders, 156–58

loss of. See Appetite, changes in, 175–76; Ascariasis, 15; Depression, 54–55; Diabetes mellitus, 55–57; Hepatitis, 78–79; Influenza, 93–94; Lupus erythematosus, 102–3; Lyme disease, 103–4; Malabsorption syndrome, 106; Phynelketonuria, 120–21; Rabies, 129; Regional enteritis, 129; Tapeworms, 154; Tuberculosis, 162–63

Armpits, swollen lymph nodes in. See Hodgkin's disease, 84–85; Infectious mononucleosis, 92–93.

with pain. See AIDS, 4–6

scaly crusts on. See Cradle cap, 49

Attention span, short, 176–77

Back, rigid muscles and. See Tetanus, 155–56

one side more prominent than other. See Scoliosis, 138–39

pain in, with fever. See Kidney diseases, 98–99; Poliomyelitis, 126

tightness of, after eating. See Chinese restaurant syndrome, 42

Backache, 178–79. See also Influenza, 93–94; Menstrual difficulties, 245–46; Rabies, 129

Barking. See Tourette's syndrome, 161–62

Behavior, aggressive, 174–75. See also Depression, 54–55; Type A behavior, 278–79

bizarre. See Hypoglycemia, 89

changes in, 181–82. See also Addiction, warning signs of, 173–74

compulsive, 199

regressive, 259

Belly button, bulge below. See Hernia, 79–81

Blackheads. See Acne, 3–4

Bladder, control of. See Bed-wetting, 179–81; Encephalitis, 63–64

seizures and, 139–41

Bleeding, from bowels. See Blood in stools, 182–83; Measles, 107–8

from mouth. See Measles, 107–8

from nose. See Measles, 107–8; Rheumatic fever, 132–33

uncontrollable. See Hemophilia, 77–78

Blinking, lapse of consciousness and. See Seizure disorders, 139–41

involuntary. See Tics, 158; Tourette's syndrome, 161–62

Blisters, 29–30. See also Eczema, 62–63

on eyes. See Herpes simplex, 81–82

on feet. See Athlete's foot, 17–18

Blisters (*cont.*)
  on genitals. See Herpes simplex,
    81–82
  on lips. See Cold sore, 44–45; Herpes
    simplex, 81–82
  in mouth. See Herpangina, 81;
    Herpetic stomatitis, 82
  oozing, crusts and. See Impetigo, 91
  red, dotted, and joining together. See
    Heat rash, 74–75
  with rash, and itching. See Poison ivy,
    125; Scabies, 137–38
    on one side of body. See Herpes
      Zoster, 82
  with redness, from sun exposure. See
    Sunburn, 151
Blood, clotting problem with. See
    Hemophilia, 77–78
  in newborn's eye. See Birth injuries,
    23–25
  from nipples. See Breasts, conditions
    of, 32–34
  in stools, 182–83. See also Amebic
    dysentery, 8–9; Anal fissure,
    9–10; Bacillary dysentery, 21;
    Bowel movement, abnormal,
    189–90; Colitis, 45
  on toilet paper. See Anal fissure, 9–10
  in vaginal discharge. See Vaginitis,
    165
Blood pressure, low, 89. See also
    Anaphylactic shock, 10–11;
    Anorexia nervosa, 12–13
Blue, turning color of. See Breath
    holding, 192–93; Croup, 49–51;
    Heart, hole in, 85; Pertussis,
    118–20; Pneumonia, 123–24;
    Septicemia, 141
  seizures and, 139–41
Body, hot to the touch, after sun
    exposure. See Sunstroke, 152
Bowel movement, accidental. See Fecal
    soiling, 216–17
  bloody, 182–83. See also
    Intussusception, 95
  difficulty with. See Bowel movement,
    abnormal, 189–90; Constipation,
    200; Hernia, 79–81
  loss of control of. See Encephalitis,
    63–64
  seizures and, 139–41
Brain, damage to. See Phenylketonuria,
    120–121

Breasts, conditions of, 32–33
  development of. See Sexual
    development, premature, 262
Breath, holding of, 192–93
  foul odor of, 179
  shortness of. See Anemia, 11–12;
    Bites, snake, 26–28; Bites, spider,
    28; Laryngitis, 101;
    Pneumothorax, 124; Thyroid
    disorders, 156–58
Breathing, arrest of. See Reye's
    syndrome, 130–31; Sudden infant
    death syndrome, 150–51
  decreased rate in. See Septicemia, 141
  difficulty with. See Anaphylactic
    shock, 10–11; Ascariasis, 15;
    Asthma, 15; Bites, snake, 26–28;
    Bites, spider, 28; Botulism, 31–
    32; Croup, 49–51; Cystic fibrosis,
    51–52; Diabetes mellitus, 55–57;
    Diphtheria, 58–59; Hay fever, 73;
    Hernia, 79–81; Laryngitis, 101;
    Pertussis, 118–20; Pneumonia,
    123–24; Poliomyelitis, 126; Rh
    problems, 131–32; Rheumatic
    fever, 132–33; Tonsillitis, 160–61;
    Tuberculosis, 162–63
  after animal bite. See Bites, snake,
    26–28; Bites, spider, 28; Rabies,
    129
  with rigid chest. See Tetanus,
    155–56
  after sun exposure. See Sunstroke,
    152
  increased rate in. See Bronchiolitis,
    34; Hyperventilation, 88–89;
    Panic attack, 117
  irregular. See Intestinal obstruction,
    94–95
  noisy. See Croup, 49–51; Pertussis,
    118–20; Pneumonia, 123–24
  shallow. See Heat stroke, 75;
    Immunization reaction, 234–36;
    Pneumonia, 123–24; Shock,
    142–43
Bruising, proneness to. See Cancer,
    37–39; Hemophilia, 77–78;
    Leukemia, 101–2
Bulge, beneath skin. See Hernia, 79–81
Bumps, on newborn's head. See Birth
    injuries, 23–25
  purple, under the skin. See AIDS, 4–6
  on skin. See Allergy, 6–8

Eyelids, abscess on (*cont.*)
swollen. See Conjunctivitis, 48
Eyestrain. See Farsightedness, 66;
Nearsightedness, 115

Face, malformation of. See Down's
syndrome, 59–60
puffiness of. See Thyroid disorders,
156–58
reddish marks on. See Hemangioma,
75–77
spastic grimacing of. See Tics, 158;
Tourette's syndrome, 161–62
tightening muscles of. See Teeth
grinding, 272–73
Faintness. See Panic attack, 117; Reye's
syndrome, 130–31
clamminess and. See Anaphylactic
shock, 10–11
Fatigue. See Addiction, warning signs of,
173–74; AIDS, 4–6; Behavior,
changes in, 181–82; Diabetes
mellitus, 55–57; Encephalitis,
63–64; Hypoglycemia, 89;
Infectious mononucleosis, 92–93;
Influenza, 93–94; Leukemia,
101–2; Rabies, 129; Rheumatic
fever, 132–33; Thyroid disorders,
156–58
Fear. See Panic attack, 117
Feathers, sensitivity to. See Hay fever, 73
Fever. See Temperature, high
Fontanel, bulging. See Meningitis,
109–10
Food, preoccupation with. See Anorexia
nervosa, 12–13; bulimia, 36
Foot, curved, hooked. See Toeing in,
159–60
twisted. See Clubfoot, 44
Forehead, reddish area on. See
Hemangioma, 75–77
spastic wrinkling of. See Tics, 158
Frustration. See Attention-deficit
disorders, 18–19; Attention span,
short, 176–77; Depression, 54–55
Fur, sensitivity to. See Allergy, 6–8

Gas, excess of, 223; Lactase deficiency/
lactose intolerance, 240–41;
Malabsorption syndrome, 106;
Milk allergy, 110–11
Glands, swollen. See Hodgkin's disease,
84–85; Infectious mononucleosis,

92–93; Juvenile rheumatoid
arthritis, 96–97; Lymphangitis,
104–5; Rubella, 135–36
after immunization. See Immunization
reaction, 234–36
in neck/jaw. See Mumps, 112
with sore throat/fever. See Strep
throat, 149
Goiter. See Thyroid disorders, 156–58
Grasses, sensitivity to. See Hay fever,
73
Groin, bulging of. See Hernia, 79–81
rash in. See Jock itch, 96
swollen lymph nodes in. See Hodgkin's
disease, 84–85; Infectious
mononucleosis, 92–93
Growth, abnormal. See Juvenile
rheumatoid arthritis, 96–97;
Thyroid disorders, 156–58
failure of, 223–24. See also
Malabsorption syndrome, 106
Growths (tumors). See Cancer
on hands/feet. See Warts, 167
Grunting, uncontrollable. See Tourette's
syndrome, 161–62
Gurgling sound. See Seizure disorders,
139–41

Hair, abnormal growth of. See Anorexia
nervosa, 12–13; Sexual
development, premature, 262
animal, sensitivity to. See Allergy, 6–8;
Hay fever, 73
dry and dull. See Thyroid disorders,
156–58
flakes in. See Dandruff, 203
loss of, 225. See also Ringworm,
134–35
plucking of. See Hair, loss of, 225
Hallucinations. See Hypoglycemia, 89
with fever. See Encephalitis, 63–64
Hand washing. See Compulsive behavior,
199
Hands, puffiness. See Thyroid disorders,
156–58
Head, banging of, 226. See also Autism,
19–20; Ear infections, 61–62
flattened, small. See Down's syndrome,
59–60
soft sport, bulging. See Meningitis,
109–10
sudden drop to chest. See Seizure
disorders, 139–41